EKG/ECG Interpretation

Everything You Need to Know About the 12-Lead EKG/ECG Interpretation and How to Diagnose and Treat Arrhythmias

DAVID ANDERSSON

Contents

Contents

Contents

Contents

Contents

Contents

Introduction

Learning the ECG is a valuable skill for both medical practitioners and non-practitioners. Knowing how to interpret ECG readings will help with understanding how specific features of a person's heart can affect him or her. This knowledge will guide appropriate care, and prevent undesirable complications from happening.

This book is intended to be a beginner's guide that will provide a mental framework for more advanced topics. Reading this is enough for you to comprehend ECG readings, but you need to know as much as you can so that you can provide the best care.

Study this book and other materials thoroughly. If there is something you do not understand, seek clarification before moving on to something else, to minimize your confusion. The more you understand something, the better you will be able to respond to it - especially during emergencies.

Aside from this, reading from an introductory book may not prepare you enough for the diversity of ECG readings. You need to practice reading as many ECG strips as possible while knowing the patients' symptoms and diagnosis. This will consolidate everything you will learn from this book and other learning materials.

Each chapter includes exercises. The answers for these are found at the end of the book. Answering these will serve as your review for the chapter.

With that being said, let us begin with the basics of ECG - what it is, what it does, and what you need to prepare for it.

Chapter 1:

The Basics

The electrocardiogram (ECG or EKG) is a device that detects the electrical activity of the heart in order for heart problems to be diagnosed. It displays this as line tracings that are printed on paper.

An ECG and an EKG is one and the same. The German translation for electrocardiogram is elektro-kardiographie, which is shortened to EKG.

An ECG/EKG has numerous uses:

- » It determines the heart's electrical activity
- » It finds the cause/s of pressure or pain within the chest
- » It uncovers the reasons for heart disease symptoms
- » It checks whether the heart chamber walls are abnormally thick
- » It evaluates the effects of medicines and heart implants
- » It examines heart health

When combined with special algorithms (calculations), this device can study numerous biometrics (measurements related to a person's biology), as follows:

- » Heart rate
- » Heart rate variability

» Heart age

» Breathing index

» Fatigue

» Stress

Although the ECG gives us several details about the heart, it cannot predict if the person will have a heart attack or when it will happen. It may not adequately pick up heart problems; someone with heart disease may have a normal EKG. Because of this, the doctors will also look at other factors such as the medical history, other symptoms present, physical examinations, and additional tests.

Sometimes, a problematic EKG output only registers during exercise, scenarios when the heart is stressed, or while the patient is currently experiencing the symptoms. For these instances, ambulatory (walking) and stress EKGs are done.

An EKG done while a person is having a heart attack may seem normal or the same as his/her previous EKGs. When this happens, the EKG is repeated over a period of time, such as over several hours or a few days to detect significant changes. These are labelled as serial EKGs.

ECG Procedure

Before taking an ECG/EKG, the patient will be asked to do the following:

» Report all medicines taken – these may affect how the tests will turn out.

» Take off all jewellery from the neck, the arms, and the wrists.

» Refrain from moving or talking.

» Breathe normally and relax.

» Avoid removing the electrodes before the test is done.

During the procedure, the patient will lie on the table or bed. The chest, arms, and legs may be shaved to obtain suitable surfaces for the electrodes.

The electrodes are attached to the patient's skin, at specific points on the body where cardiac electrical activity is detected. These are linked to the machine that prints the output.

The device will then record the activity for a few minutes. The patient is asked to refrain from moving too much or talking, to prevent interfering with the readings.

When the reading is obtained, the electrodes are removed from the body and the paste is wiped off from the skin. The patient then gets up from the bed or table.

ECG Tools

There are certain instruments that help with ECG interpretation:

Calipers

Calipers are perhaps the most important tool in ECG interpretation. To use one, put one pointed edge against one end of what you are measuring, and the other edge at the other end. The caliper will maintain this position. You can then move on to a blank area of the ECG strip. Count the number of boxes to get your measurements (example: 1 small box = 0.04 seconds, 1 big box = 0.20 seconds, and so on).

You can use calipers to check whether the distance between complexes is equal. Measure the complex with the two pins. Hold the right pin down and gently swing the left pin to the next complex. If they are the same, the next complex will coincide with the pin. This technique is called "walking", and it is useful for determining complex regularity and detecting ECG abnormalities.

Aside from width, calipers can also measure wave heights. You can likewise "walk" the caliper, so that you will know the biggest or smallest complexes and see whether a wave is more positive or more negative.

ECG Ruler

This helps with measuring ECG, but it is not that necessary, since a caliper can do what this does.

Axis-wheel Rulers

Axis-wheel rulers are used to calculate waves and segments' true axis. This ruler has a red line and a perpendicular arrow.

Straight edge

It evaluates the baseline, and can determine elevations and depressions.

At first, you may be dependent on these instruments, which can enable you to make accurate diagnoses. After a lot of practice, you will be able to quickly make measurements without having to use them.

Calibration

The end of an ECG strip will usually have a calibration box, which is 10 mm high and 0.20 seconds wide. This says that the ECG follows the standard format. This has a rate of 25 mm/sec.

There are ECGs that have a half-standard calibration, especially when the complexes are so large that they overlap. When this is the case, the calibration box will have a stair-like design.

The third calibration is set at 50 mm/sec. The calibration box is 0.40 seconds in width.

It is important to check the calibration of the ECG, in order to evaluate the tracings correctly.

These are some of the basic things you need to know before diving into the details of ECG interpretation.

The next chapters will tackle the heart and the mechanisms of the heartbeat so that you will understand how they affect the ECG readings.

Exercises

1. What does ECG mean?

    a. Electric Cardiology Gadget

    b. Electrocardiogram

    c. Electrocartographer

    d. Electrode Cardiograph

2. All of these are uses of ECG except one, which is it?

    a. Monitors the heart's electrical activity

    b. Finds the cause of chest pain

    c. Predicts heart attacks

    d. Evaluates heart health

3. True or False: Stress and ambulatory tests are done to know how the heart behaves while in its normal state.

4. A device that has pointed edges and can be used to get measurements by "walking"

    a. ECG ruler

    b. straight edge

    c. axis-wheel ruler

    d. caliper

5. A calibration box 10 mm high and 0.20 seconds wide has a rate of _75_ mm/sec

6. A _ calibration has a stair-like design.

7. The third calibration is set at _ mm/sec and is .40 seconds in width.

8. It is important to check the calibration of the ECG to determine the _ of the tracings.

    a. height

    b. voltage

    c. rate

    d. form

9. Several ECGs done over a period of time are called _ ECGs

    a. multiple

    b. comparative

    c. serial

    d. secondary

10. True or false: The patient needs to be sedated during the procedure to get a clear reading.

Chapter 2:

The Heart

To understand the ECG better, it is helpful to study the heart itself. Without this foundational knowledge, the ECG may become undecipherable.

The heart is in the center of the chest, slightly tilting downwards to the left. It is nearer the front of the body than the back.

The heart functions as a pump with four main chambers, with two atria (plural for atrium) and two ventricles. The left ventricle releases blood into the peripheral circulatory system (the blood vessels of the body), while the right ventricle pumps blood into the pulmonary system (lungs).

Oxygen-rich blood from the heart passes through the arteries, while oxygen-depleted blood from the body returns to the heart through the veins.

After oxygen is used by the body cells, the blood is returned to the heart. The right ventricle pushes this through the pulmonary artery and into the lungs, where it is infused with oxygen again. This flows into the left ventricle, which pumps the blood through the aorta and into the blood vessels of the entire body.

The right ventricle takes up most of the front part of the heart, but the left ventricle is the one that produces most of the electricity.

Electrical Conduction

The heart has cells that are designed to conduct electricity – some of them are responsible for setting a pace, while others transmit electrical impulses. This is an electro-chemical process that happens in the myocardium (heart muscles) found in the walls of the heart.

The atrial myocytes (heart muscle cells) activate each other in sequence. The intermodal pathways carry the impulse from the sino-atrial (SA) node to the atrioventricular (AV) node, reaching the Purkinje system, which goes around the ventricles and energizes the myocardial cells.

These cells set the pace at which the heart beats. All cells in the conduction system can create a pace, but the rate of each cell type is slower than the rate of those that came before it. Thus, the SA node has the fastest pace; the AV node has the second fastest, and so on, with the last component having the slowest pace. The node with the fastest rate establishes the rate because it resets all the paces of those that come after it. If it malfunctions, the next fastest will serve as its backup, ensuring that the heart beats at near the normal rate.

These are the approximate rates of each component:

- » SA node cells: 60-100 BPM (beats per minute)
- » Atrial cells: 55-60 BPM
- » AV node: 45-50 BPM
- » Bundle of His cells: 40-45 BPM
- » Bundle branch cells: 40-45 BPM
- » Purkinje cells: 20-40 BPM

SA Node

Found in the wall of the right atrium, the SA node is the main pacemaker.

Internodal Pathways

The anterior, middle, and posterior pathways (located in the right atrium and inter-atrial septum - the wall separating the two atria) send the pacing impulses from the SA node towards the AV node. This pathway also consists of the Bachmann bundle, which carries impulses through the inter-atrial septum.

The AV node

Within the right atrium and near the coronary sinus, the AV node slows down the conduction of the atria to the ventricles, to enable atrial contraction to occur. Slowing down the pace enables the atria to fill the ventricles, and maximizes the output of the heart.

The Bundle of His

The Bundle of His begins at the AV node, and splits into the left and right bundle branches. It is partially located in the right atrium walls and in the interventricular septum, which is the partition between the ventricles. This allows for transmission of impulses between the ventricles and atria.

The Left Bundle Branch

The LBB originates from the end of the His bundle, traverses the interventricular septum, and ends at the start of the left anterior and left posterior fascicles (LAF and LPF). This innervates the left ventricle, and the left part of the interventricular septum.

The Right Bundle Branch

This also begins at the His bundle, but it innervates the right ventricle and right part of the interventricular septum. It ends at the Purkinje fibres.

The Left Anterior Fascicle (LAF)

The LAF goes through the left ventricle, and reaches the Purkinje cells that energize the front and top parts of the left ventricle. This consists of a single strand.

The Left Posterior Fascicle (LPF)

The LPF is composed of many strands that lead to the Purkinje cells, that innervate the back and bottom part of the left ventricle.

The Purkinje System

This is composed of cells beneath the inner layer of the heart (myocardium). These directly innervate the cells of the myocardium, and start the ventricular depolarization cycle.

Electrolytes

Electrolytes enable cells to generate electricity. They affect how the heart beats, so you need to have an idea of how they work to interpret an ECG well.

Each cell of the heart (myocardial cell/myocyte) is made of two parts that glide over each other. These partitions are linked to the outside of the cells, and they are made up of myosin molecules that are distributed between actin molecules.

The cells are linked together to create long bands called myofibrils, which in turn are linked together by connective tissue to create fluid-covered sheets. The bands expand and contract according to the electrical impulse that reaches them.

When one or all of the bands in a sheet contract, the sheet shortens. It returns to its original size when all of the bands expand. These sheets form the chambers of the heart: the 2 atria on top and the 2 ventricles at the bottom. The atria are smaller and thinner than the ventricles below them.

Each cell has fluid inside and outside of it - this contains water, proteins, and salts. When the salts interact with fluid, they break down into particles that have either a positive and negative charge - these are called ions. The positively charged ions, or cations, are potassium, sodium, and calcium while the negatively charged ions (anions) are mostly chloride.

Action potential of cardiac muscles

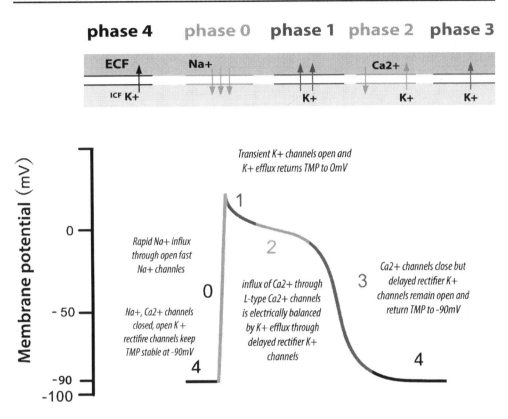

Figure 1. Impulse transmission in heart muscle cells

A living cell maintains a difference between the concentrations of the ions, and charges within the cell and outside it. Normally, the inside of the cell has a higher concentration of potassium, while the outside environment has a higher sodium concentration. There is a negative charge within the cell as compared to outside, because calcium, a positively charged ion, also floats outside the cell.

The difference between electrical charges within and outside of the cell wall is considered as the cell's electrical potential. Because ions and chargers tend to maintain neutrality, sodium tends to enter the cell wall and potassium tends to exit. In order to maintain its electrical potential, the cell has mechanisms that control these ions in ways that do not allow them to follow their natural tendency.

Phase 4 (Resting Potential)

The sodium-potassium ATPase pump facilitates the movement of ions around the cell, to protect the electrical charge and concentration. It uses ATP to push out three sodium ions, and pull in two potassium ions. This results in a greater positive charge existing on the outside of the cell as compared to the inside. Because of this, the resting myocyte's electrical potential is maintained from between -70 to -90 millivolts.

After a while, the ions begin to overload the pump, and the cell's interior becomes less negative because more sodium ions are entering.

Threshold potential

Gradually, the cell becomes positively charged, and this opens up a new batch of channels – the fast sodium channels. These are one-way valves that permit only ions such as sodium to enter the cell.

Phase 0

When these valves open, sodium ions rapidly enter the cell and cause a surge of positive charge inside it. This impulse stimulates the cell, and passes on to the cells near it, until all cells have been activated.

Depolarization

When the cell is no longer negatively charged or polarized, it is now said to be depolarized, and it is also positive like the fluids outside it.

Phase 1

When the cell reaches its maximum positive charge, it enters phase 1 of the action potential. This triggers chloride ions (negative charge) to enter the cell, which slows down the entrance of sodium ions (positive charge).

Phase 2

The rapid sodium channels close down at this point, while the slow sodium channels and the calcium channels open. The slow sodium channels let sodium ions slowly enter the cell, while the calcium channels let calcium enter. Since calcium has two positive charges, it helps maintain the cell's depolarized state.

Calcium helps cells contract by triggering actin and myosin proteins to move against each other. When there is more calcium, the proteins clamp faster and contract longer.

Phase 3

A few potassium channels open to make potassium ions exit the cell, causing rapid repolarization. The negative charge of the cell returns as positively charged potassium leaves it. This leads to the resting potential (phase 4) and the cycle begins again.

Each cell of the heart has these action potential cycles, and can polarize and depolarize 70-100 times in one minute. Even though there are millions of cells in the heart, they all act together because of the electrical conduction system. These electrical discharges come together and create one large current or electrical axis. The ECG picks up these electrical potentials and transforms them into patterns.

It is better if you understand what has been discussed in this chapter before you move on to the next ones. Doing so will help you integrate the information more easily.

Exercises

1. The _ pumps blood through the aorta and into the blood vessels of the body.

    a. Left atrium

    b. Right atrium

    c. Left ventricle

    d. Right ventricle

2. The _ takes up most of the front part of the heart.

    a. Left atrium

    b. Right atrium

    c. Left ventricle

    d. Right ventricle

3. The _ produces most of the electrical activity of the heart.

    a. Left atrium

    b. Right atrium

    c. Left ventricle

    d. Right ventricle

4. The main pacemaker of the heart is:

    a. SA Node

    b. AV Node

    c. Bundle Branches

    d. Ventricles

5. The secondary pacemaker of the heart is:

    a. SA Node

    b. AV Node

    c. Bundle Branches

    d. Ventricles

6. Which of the following transmits electrical impulses between the SA and AV nodes?

    a. SA Node

    b. AV Node

    c. Bundle Branches

    d. Ventricles

7. The SA node has a rate of _.

    a. 120 - 200 BPM

    b. 60 - 100 BPM

    c. 40 – 60 BPM

    d. 20 – 40 BPM

8. The main negative ion is:

    a. Sodium

    b. Potassium

    c. Chloride

    d. Calcium

9. There is a high concentration of _ inside a cell and a high concentration of _ outside it.

    a. Potassium, Sodium

    b. Sodium, Potassium

    c. Calcium, Magnesium

    d. Magnesium, Calcium

10. The ion that enables the troponin and tropomyosin in heart tissue to clamp together.

    a. Potassium

    b. Sodium

    c. Magnesium

    d. Calcium

Chapter 3:

The ECG Complex

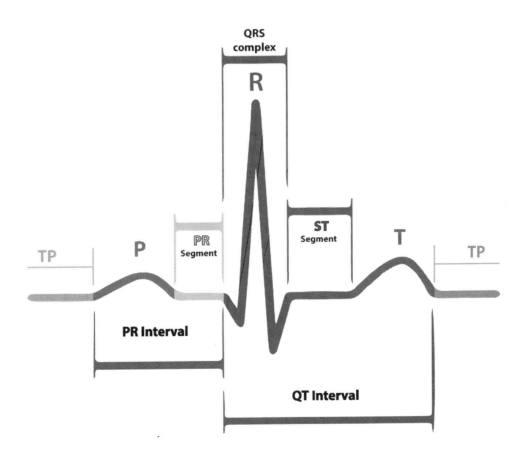

Figure 2. Components of the ECG complex

The ECG records waves, intervals, and segments. These have particular morphologies (forms), axes, durations, and amplitudes when normal. When the ECG readings are different from these traits, there may be something wrong with the heart.

A wave represents a cardiac event, such as atrial depolarization, atrial repolarization, ventricular depolarization, ventricular repolarization, and His bundle transmission.

A wave is a deflection from a baseline, which is the line from one TP segment to another one next to it. It can be single, positive, negative, biphasic, isolated, or have multiple parts that can be positive or negative.

An interval is the time distance between two cardiac events. A segment is a specific part of a complex on an ECG. A segment is different from an interval.

This is the normal sequence of the waves:

» The P wave is the first positive (upward) deflection that shows up on the ECG

» The Q wave is the first negative (downward) wave, which appears after the P wave

» The R wave is the first positive wave after the Q wave

» The S wave is the first negative wave after R wave

» The T wave is a positive wave that appears after the S wave.

Tall waves are given big letters, while small waves are labelled with small letters.

Prime waves

Waves are called prime when they cross the baseline, or change directions.

When there are extra waves where they aren't supposed to be, they are labelled as prime waves.

A wave can be a double prime when it occurs twice.

The P Wave

The P wave is normally the first wave on the TP segment. It represents the atria's electrical depolarization. The wave begins when the SA node fires, and it embodies the impulse transmission through the internodal pathways, the Bachmann bundle, and the atrial myocytes.

Since the P wave represents atrial depolarization, P wave abnormalities signify atrial abnormalities. Check the inferior leads (II, III, and aVF), and precordial lead V1 for this.

The wave duration is between 0.08 – 0.11 seconds, or less than 120 ms. Its axis is commonly directed downwards, and to the left (Axis: 0 to 75 degrees), since it goes through the atrioventricular node and atrial appendages.

The first one third of the wave embodies the right atrial activation, the last third represents the left atrial activation, and the middle is the blend between the two.

P waves are normally upright in leads I and II and inverted in lead aVR. They are monophasic in lead II and biphasic in V1.

In V1, the P wave is biphasic and begins with a positive deflection, showing right atrial activation, and ends with a negative deflection, which reflects left atrial activation. Because of this, the state of each individual atrium can be determined by looking at each part of this waveform.

These are some things that can be known from P waves:

> » Tall and prolonged P waves can indicate atrial enlargement.
> » Bifid P waves (broad and notched) are associated with left atrial enlargement, while peaked P waves are linked to right atrial enlargement.
> » Inverted P waves indicate ectopic atrial and junctional rhythms.
> » Variable P wave forms hint to multifocal atrial rhythms.

The TP Wave

The TP wave symbolizes the repolarization of the atria. This moves in the opposite direction of the P wave.

This is not commonly obvious because it coincides with the more prominent QRS wave.

The TP wave appears when the QRS is absent, such as in the case of AV dissociation or non-conducted beats. This also shows up in PR depression, or in the ST segment depression during sinus tachycardia.

It shows as ST depression because the QRS arrives earlier and the TP wave draws the ST segment down.

The PR segment

The PR segment is found when the P wave ends, and the QRS complex begins. It normally lies along the baseline, but can be depressed or elevated by up to 0.8 mm. PR segment abnormalities indicate atrial infarctions/ ischemia and pericarditis.

The PR segment shows the transmission of the electrical depolarization impulse through the AV node, bundle of His, bundle branches, and Purkinje system.

The PR Interval

The PR Interval is the time period from the P wave's beginning to the QRS complex's beginning. It consists of the P wave and the PR segment.

The PR interval involves events from the start of the electrical impulse in the SA node to ventricular depolarization. (Beginning of impulse, atrial depolarization and repolarization, stimulation of AV node, His bundle, bundle branch, and Purkinje System).

This normally lasts from 0.12 – 0.20 seconds.

If it's longer than 0.20 seconds, it is a sign of a first-degree AV block.

It can also be called as PQ interval when a Q wave begins the QRS complex.

The QRS Complex

The QRS complex reflects ventricular depolarization. It usually lasts 0.06 – 0.11 seconds with an axis of -30 to +105 degrees, going downward and to the left.

It has two or more waves which have their own name.

The Q wave is usually the first negative deflection after the P wave, but it can sometimes be absent.

The R wave is the first positive deflection after the P wave. It can be the starting wave of the QRS complex if the Q is not around.

The first negative deflection following the R wave is the S wave.

Q Wave

A Q wave is considered significant if it lasts for 0.03 seconds or longer, or if it is as tall or taller than 1/3 of the R wave. When these conditions are present, there is a myocardial infarction (MI).

Insignificant Q waves are traditionally found in I, aVl and V6, and these are caused by septal innervations. These are usually called septal Qs.

Intrinsicoid Deflection

This begins from the start of the QRS complex to the start of the downward slope of the R wave, in leads that begin with an R wave and do not have a Q wave. It symbolizes the time taken for the electrical impulse to traverse the Purkinje system from within the inner layer to outer layer of the heart.

It is shorter in the right precordial leads (V1-V2) because the right ventricle is thinner than the left.

The intrinsicoid deflection will be longer if the myocardium is thicker than normal (eg. Ventricular hypertrophy), or when the electrical system conducts slower in that area because of a delay (eg. Left bundle branch block).

These are the upper normal limits for intrinsicoid deflection:

> » Left precordials = 0.045 seconds
> » Right precordials = 0.035 seconds

The ST segment

The ST segment is the electrically neutral period in between ventricular depolarization and repolarization. In this phase, the myocardium is maintaining its contraction to push the blood from the ventricles. Its axis is normally inferior and to the left.

This is the section from the QRS complex's end to the T wave's start. It is usually found on the baseline, but can deviate up to 1 mm from it in normal patients' limb leads, and 3 mm in the right precordials. This may be caused by left ventricular hypertrophy or an early repolarization pattern.

The J point marks the spot where the QRS complex stops and the ST segment begins.

When the ST segment is elevated, it should be considered as significant, as it can reveal a myocardial infarction or injury.

The T Wave

The T wave signifies ventricular repolarization. This is the next positive or negative deflection after the ST segment. It is expected to begin in the same direction as that of the QRS complex. The axis is downward and to the left for this wave as well.

The T wave is asymmetrical, with the first part dropping or rising slowly and the last part moving rapidly.

To check whether the T wave is symmetrical or not, draw a perpendicular line from the wave's peak to the baseline and compare the two sides.

Symmetric Ts usually signify problems.

The QT Interval

The QT interval comprises of the QRS complex, ST segment, and T wave.

It involves cardiac events of ventricular systole, that is, from the start of ventricular depolarization until the end of the repolarization cycle.

The QT interval depends on the patient's age, sex, heart rate, and electrolyte condition.

A prolonged QT can mean arrhythmias.

QTc means QT corrected interval. This is adjusted according to the heart rate. As heart rate increases, the QT interval shortens, and as the heart rate decreases, so the QT interval would lengthen as well.

To obtain QTc, add QT + 1.75 * (ventricular rate -60)

The QTc interval normally lasts 0.410 seconds, and anything longer than .419 is considered prolonged.

The U wave

The U wave is the small wave commonly seen after the T wave and before the following P wave. This has low voltage, and has the same direction as the T wave.

It is not clear as to what it symbolizes, but it is theorized that it stands for ventricular depolarization and endocardial repolarization.

It is seen in normal individuals especially those with bradycardia (slow heartbeats). It is also evident in hypokalemia or low potassium in the blood, thus there is no hyperkalemia (high levels of potassium) when a U wave exists.

The R-R Interval

The R-R interval is the distance between two identical points or peaks of two consecutive QRS complexes.

This is used to determine whether the rhythm is regular or irregular. Those with regular rhythms have consistent R-R intervals.

The P-P interval

This is the distance between two identical points on a P wave, and the next one. This is used to assess rhythm abnormalities such as atrial flutter, Wenckeback second-degree heart block and third-degree heart block.

Baseline

The baseline of the ECG is the line from the TP of one complex to the TP of another one.

The PR segment should be on this line, but there are times when it is elevated.

Exercises

1. Which of the following represents atrial depolarization

    a. P Wave

    b. TP Wave

    c. QRS Complex

    d. T Wave

    e. U Wave

2. Which of the following represents atrial repolarization

    a. P Wave

    b. TP Wave

    c. QRS Complex

    d. T Wave

    e. U Wave

3. Which of the following represents ventricular depolarization

    a. P Wave

    b. TP Wave

    c. QRS Complex

    d. T Wave

    e. U Wave

4. Which of the following represents ventricular repolarization

   a. P Wave

   b. TP Wave

   c. QRS Complex

   d. T Wave

   e. U Wave

5. Which of the following is theorized to represent endocardial repolarization

   a. P Wave

   b. TP Wave

   c. QRS Complex

   d. T Wave

   e. U Wave

6. A line between a TP segment of one complex to the TP segment of the following complex is called:

   a. Baseline

   b. P-P Interval

   c. Q-T Interval

   d. ST Segment

7. Interval representing all cardiac events of ventricular systole.

    a. Baseline

    b. P-P Interval

    c. Q-T Interval

    d. ST Segment

8. A Q wave with a height that is one third or greater of the R wave, and lasts longer than 0.03 seconds is:

    a. Normal Sinus Rhythm

    b. Benign Arrhythmia

    c. A Myocardial Infarction sign

    d. Bradycardia

9. Which of the following symbolizes the time it takes for the electrical impulse to traverse the Purkinje system that runs along the inner to the outer layer of the heart.

    a. P-P interval

    b. R-R interval

    c. ST segment

    d. Intrinsicoid Deflection

10. The distance between two identical peaks of consecutive QRS complexes is known as:

    a. P-P interval

    b. R-R interval

    c. ST segment

    d. Intrinsicoid Deflection

Chapter 4

Making Interpretations

Interpreting the ECG take some practice, because there's a lot going on in the graph. It is important that you understand everything you read here. You don't have to memorize everything, but do keep notes, or this book handy.

When you have an ECG to interpret, look at it broadly and take note of any outstanding features. Do not dwell on the tiny details at this point, but try to form a general impression about it. Does it seem like a case of arrhythmia, ischemia, etc.? Keep your tentative conclusion in mind as you go through the next steps.

An ECG gives a lot of information that is only unlocked if you know what each part of the tracings mean. In general, a normal reading has the following characteristics:

> » The heart beat is somewhere from 60 to 100 beats per minute (for adults)
>
> » It shows a regular rhythm
>
> » The tracing follows the normal pattern (this will be discussed later)
>
> » A reading is considered abnormal when these are present:
>
> » The heart beat is faster than average (above 100 BPM)
>
> » It is slower than normal (below 60 BPM)

» It displays an irregular rhythm

» The tracing deviates from the expected outline

After gaining an overview, go over the ECG sequentially. Determine where the normal and abnormal beats are. For the normal ones, evaluate the axis, intervals, blocks, and other things you need to find out. For the abnormal beats, think about what may be causing them.

Before anything else, you must know that the above features are just general indicators of normality and abnormality.

If you want to get useful insights, you have to consider other features. Read on to know how to get specific information from ECG readings.

Heart Rate

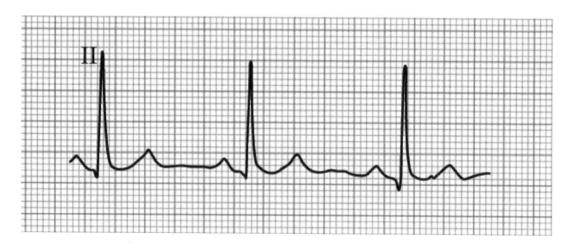

The ECG paper has tiny boxes that measure 1 mm each, and these are grouped together to form bigger boxes. It runs under the pen at 25 mm/sec, thus each box on the graph represents 1/25th of a second, or 0.04 seconds).

The large boxes have 5 small boxes each. Each one represents 5 x 0.04 seconds = 0.2 seconds.

5 large boxes mean 5 x 0.2 seconds, which is equal to 1 second.

In summary:

> » 1 small box (1 mm) = 0.04 seconds
>
> » 1 large box (5 mm) = 5 small boxes = 0.2 seconds
>
> » 5 large boxes (25 mm)= 1 second

The ECG is traditionally 10 seconds long, with each lead covering 2.5 seconds. The paper has three to four strips. The top three strips have 12 leads.

Bear in mind that the vertical height of a segment or wave is measured by millimetres, while the width is measured in milliseconds. This is because the width of the tracing reveals the duration of the electrical activity, while the height shows its voltage.

Some ECG devices calculate the heart rate on their own, but they may be inaccurate, especially when the waveforms are abnormal. It is always better to know how to make calculations manually.

There are many ways to compute for the rate of the heartbeat:

> » For regular rhythms, count the number of large squares in one R-R interval. Divide 300 by the number of squares.
>
> » For fast rhythms, count the small squares in one R-R interval, and divide 1,500 by that number.
>
> » For slow or irregular rhythms, multiply the number of complexes by 6 to obtain the average rate of the heartbeat for every 10 seconds.

Check: is the heart rate faster or slower than expected? Again, the normal heart rate is 60-100 beats per minute, but this may vary according to the patient's age and other health conditions.

You can already make a diagnosis based on heart rate:

For adults, the normal rate is at 60 – 100 beats per minute (BPM). If the rate is greater than 100 BPM, tachycardia is present. If it is less than 60 BPM, there is bradycardia.

Children normally have faster heart rates than adults, because of their smaller body sizes. Anything faster than the values given below counts as tachycardia; if slower, then it is bradycardia.

» Newborn babies: 110 – 150 BPM

» 2 years old: 85 – 125 BPM

» 4 years old: 75 – 115 BPM

» 6 years old and older: 60 – 100 BPM

Rhythm

The heartbeat rhythm is more easily studied by using a rhythm strip, which is most often a 10 second recording from Lead II (if you used a 12 lead ECG). Look into the other leads as well, to make a more accurate diagnosis about the rhythm.

One of the easiest things to determine from the rhythm is whether it is slow or fast (bradycardia or tachycardia), and whether it's irregular or regular.

Measuring Rhythm

There are two ways to measure rhythm:

Using a piece of paper and pencil:

Place the paper along the baseline. Move it up so that the edge is near the R wave's peak. On your paper, mark the R waves of two consecutive QRS complexes to get the R-R interval. Transfer the paper across the ECG tracing and see whether the following R-R intervals line up with your marks. If yes, you can say that the ventricular rhythm is regular. If not, it is irregular. Do the same for the P waves (P-P intervals), to know whether the heart's atrial rhythm is regular or irregular.

Using calipers:

Place one point of your caliper on the peak of an R wave. Adjust the calipers so that the other point lands on the next R wave. This gives you the R-R interval. Swivel the calipers to check whether it falls on the third R wave's peak. If they do, the R-R (ventricular) rhythm is regular. If not, it is irregular. You can also determine the atrial rhythm this way, by measuring the P-P interval.

If the heartbeat has a regular rhythm, count how many complexes there are on the rhythm strip. This is usually 10 seconds long. Multiply 6 to this number to get the average number of complexes per minute.

An irregular heart rhythm may be regularly irregular, with a recurring pattern of irregularity, or irregularly irregular, which means that the rhythm is totally disorganized.

Is the rhythm grouped or ungrouped? Abnormal heart rhythms have grouped beats.

Check whether the rhythm is wide or narrow. This means observing the average width of the QRS complexes. If it is wide, there may be a conduction problem coming from the ventricles, or from the supraventricular region (above the ventricles). If narrow, the abnormality may be located in the sinus node, atria, or junctional region.

Look for P waves – if you can't find them, the patient may be experiencing atrial fibrillation or sinus arrest.

If they are present, check the ventricular and atrial rate. Are all P waves similar to each other? They are expected to be the same if there is a 1:1 conduction to the QRS complexes.

Abnormal ratios between P waves and QRS complexes may indicate atrioventricular dissociation (AV dissociation). In complete AV dissociation, the atrial and ventricular electrical activities always occur separately. In incomplete AV dissociation, capture beats show up infrequently.

If there is an abnormality in P wave shape and PR interval, this suggests that there is something wrong in the conduction of the sinus, atria, junction or ventricles. You will know the location depending on which leads the abnormalities show up.

If the heartbeat is irregular, compute for the range. Inspect the PR, QRS, QTc, PP, and RR intervals. Observe if there are irregularities in the intervals.

Consider onsets and terminations. If they are abrupt, a re-entrant process may be causing them. If gradual, it is possible that an area of the heart has increased automaticity (ability to conduct impulses).

There are a lot of heart problems that can be diagnosed by heart rhythm type:

P waves Present	Each P wave is followed by QRS complex	Sinus Node Dysfunction: Sinus bradycardia Sinus node exit block Sinus pause/arrest
	Not every P is wave followed by a QRS complex	AV Node Dysfunction: AV block: 2nd degree, Mobitz I (Wenckebach) AV block: 2nd degree, Mobitz II AV block: 2nd degree, "fixed ratio blocks" (2:1, 3:1) AV block: 2nd degree, "high grade AV block" AV block: 3rd degree (complete heart block)
P waves Absent	Broad complexes	Ventricular Escape Rhythm
	Narrow complexes	Junctional Escape Rhythm

Bradycardia

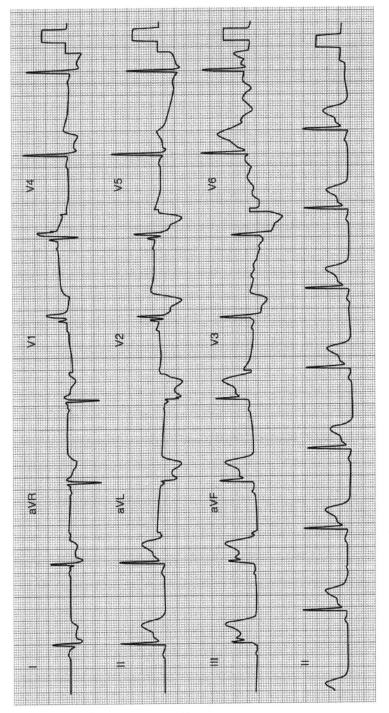

Figure 3. Sinus bradycardia: Note that the rate is about 45 bpm

Tachycardia

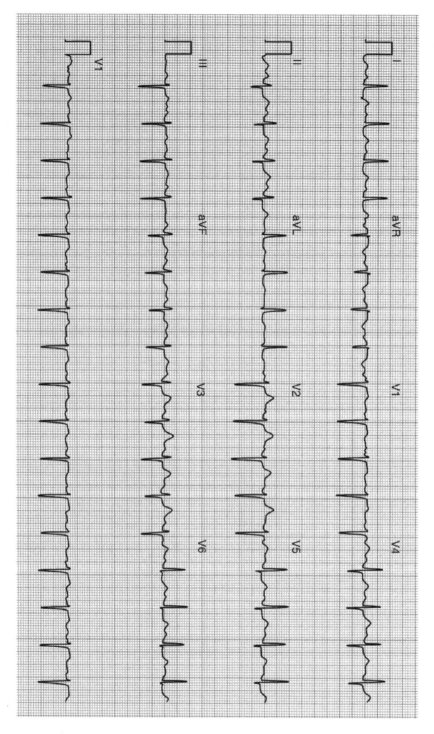

Figure 4. Sinus tachycardia: Note that rate is more than 100 bpm

Narrow QRS Complex Tachycardia/ Supraventricular Tachycardia

		Regular Rhythm	Irregular Rhythm
Atrial		Atrial Flutter Atrial Tachycardia Inappropriate Sinus Tachycardia Sinus Tachycardia Sinus node re-entrant Tachycardia	Atrial fibrillation Atrial flutter with variable block Multifocal atrial tachycardia
Atrioventricular		Automatic Junctional Tachycardia Atrioventricular re-entry Tachycardia (AVNRT) AV nodal re-entry tachycardia (AVRT)	

Broad QRS Complex Tachycardia

Regular Rhythm	Irregular Rhythm
Ventricular Tachycardia Antidromic atrioventricular re-entry tachycardia (AVRT) Any regular supraventricular tachycardia with aberrant conduction	Ventricular fibrillation Polymorphic VT Torsades de Pointes AF with Wolff-Parkinson-White syndrome Any irregular supraventricular tachycardia with aberrant conduction

Electrical Axis

Heart axis

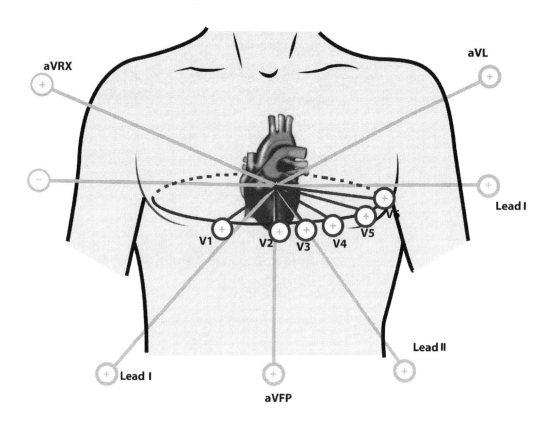

The electrical impulses are vectors which have energy and direction.

Vectors add up when they head towards the same direction, decrease in energy and change their direction when they are going in opposite locations, and add or subtract energy and change directions when they meet at an angle. The heart has numerous vectors, but as mentioned, they all combine to produce major currents. All these vectors together are referred to as the electrical axis.

There are a number of vectors detected by the ECG's electrodes: the P-wave vector, T-wave vector, ST segment vector, and QRS vector.

Electrodes pick up electrical activity. When a positive electrical impulse moves away from an electrode, the ECG registers it as a negative or downward wave. When a positive wave approaches an electrode, the ECG transforms it into a positive or upward wave. When the electrode sits at the middle of a wave, the ECG demonstrates a positive wave for the energy coming towards it, and a negative wave for the energy retreating from it.

These electrodes are placed at specific angles to the main axis, in order to get a three-dimensional view of the heart's electrical activity.

Just like with heart rate and rhythm, the electrical axis is affected by abnormalities. This is why electrical axis is studied in the ECG.

As you may recall, the QRS complex stands for ventricular depolarization. This is the strongest impulse in the heart, and thus the QRS complex determines the heart's main axis.

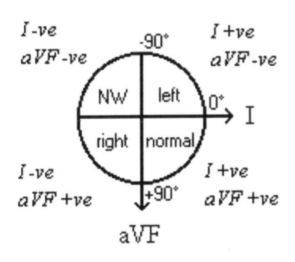

The degree of the QRS axis will tell you whether it is normal or deviated:

» Normal: between -30 to +90 degrees

» Left Axis Deviation (LAD): less than -30 degrees

» Right Axis Deviation (RAD): greater than +90 degrees

» Extreme Axis Deviation (EAD): between -90 and 180 degrees

These are some ways to determine the axis:

The quadrant method involves looking at leads I and aVF.

Lead I	Lead aVF	Quadrant	Axis
Positive	Positive	Left Lower	Normal
Positive	Negative	Left Upper	Possible LAD
Negative	Positive	Right Lower	RAD
Negative	Negative	Right Upper	EAD

The Isoelectric Lead Method is more precise than the method above, and involves finding the isoelectric/equiphasic lead. This is the frontal lead that has zero net amplitude, meaning a QRS that is a flat line or biphasic, with R wave height that is equal to Q or S wave depth.

After finding the isoelectric lead, the next step is to find the positive leads – those with the highest R waves or biggest R to S ratios.

When this is done, the QRS axis is calculated by going 90 degrees to the isoelectric lead and pointing towards the positive leads.

Later on in this book, you will know how to diagnose heart problems based on axis deviations.

Electrode Placement

Where the electrodes are placed depends on whether there are 3, 5, or 12 leads used. This book will concentrate on 12-lead ECG.

Electrodes or leads are positioned at these areas:

Limbs: Also known as extremity leads, limb leads are stationed at least 10 cm from the patient's heart. When you are using the three-lead system, it is recommended to place the leads on areas on the chest that are equally distant from the heart, instead of the limbs. The arm leads can be placed on the shoulder, at 10 cm distance from the heart..

> » Right arm (RA)
> » Left arm (LA)
> » Right leg (RL)
> » Left leg (LL)

Precordial leads: Otherwise called as chest leads, these are attached at precise points on the patient's chest.

Position V1 and V2 are located on each side of the sternum (flat bone in front of the chest) at the fourth intercostal space, or the fourth space that exists between the ribs.

To find this space, feel the Angle of Louis or the bump along the top 1/3rd portion of the sternum. This is positioned beside the second rib, and the space right below it is the second intercostal space. To find the fourth one, count two more spaces below the second.

Right after this lead is V4, placed at the fifth intercostal space. This is found at the intersection of this space and the mid-clavicular line, an imaginary line that extends downwards from the middle of the nearest clavicle (collarbone).

V3 sits in the middle of V2 and V4.

To find V5, go down, and to the right of V4. Find the intersection of this position and the anterior axillary line, or the line that extends from the front part of the armpit. Imagine a line going down from the middle of the armpit to get the mid-axillary line. This is where you place V6. .

The ECG scans the positive and negative poles of the limb electrodes to create lead I, II, and III.

Limb Leads: I, II, III, IV (aVR), V (aVL), VI (aVF)

Chest leads: V1, V2, V3, V4, V5, V6

Einthoven's Triangle

The Einthoven's Triangle is formed by the three bipolar limb leads (leads I, II, and III).

Lead I's axis runs from one shoulder to another, with the right arm (RA) lead being negative and the left arm (RA) lead being positive. Lead II's axis goes from the negative RA lead to the positive left leg (LL) lead. Lead III's axis goes from the negative left arm (LA) lead to the positive left leg (LL) lead.

Augmented Leads

Augmented leads are composed of leads aVR, aVL, and aVF. They pick up the electrical activity coming from one limb lead and one electrode. Lead aVL records input from the heart's lateral (side) wall, while lead aVF monitors input from the heart's inferior (bottom) wall. The lead aVR does not give a view to the heart but can still be useful at times.

The Hexaxial System

Hexaxial means six axes. This consists of 6 leads: I, II, III, VR, VL, and VF. The leads are 30 degrees apart from each other, thus, all 6 together encompass 180 degrees.

This system divides the heart into a back half and a front half. The positive pole of Lead I is at the right of an imaginary circle that spans this axis, while the negative pole of Lead I is at the left. The other leads also have their opposite poles on the opposite side.

Precordial System

The precordial leads on the chest are on a plane perpendicular to the hexaxial or limb leads. This system splits the heart into top and bottom parts.

>   » All these leads provide a 3-D view of the heart. Example:
>   » Anterior (front): V3 and V4
>   » Lateral (sides): I, aVl, V5, V6
>   » Septum: V1 and V2
>   » Bottom of the heart: V1, V2, aVF

Normal Sinus Rhythm (NSR)

This rhythm is present when the SA node is functioning normally as the lead pacer. The intervals should be consistent and fall within normal ranges. The rate is 60-100 BPM and regular. There is a P wave, and the P to QRS ratio is 1:1. The PR interval and QRS width are both normal. There is no grouping, and no dropped beats.

The next chapter is all about ECG abnormalities, and what to do about them. To make a diagnosis, put all of your observations together. Don't forget to include the following important details:

- » Rate
- » Rhythm
- » Axis
- » Hypertrophy
- » Interval abnormalities
- » Blocks
- » T and ST wave abnormalities

Compare the ECG findings with the patient's symptoms. Do these make sense? Is the ECG the reflection of a problem or the cause of another pre-existing health condition?

As you can see, the more you know about health, the better you can diagnose a person based on his or her ECG readings.

Exercises

1. The normal heart rate of adults is 80 - 120 BPM (True/False)

2. A normal axis is:

    a. less than -30 degrees

    b. between -90 and 180 degrees

    c. -30 to +90 degrees

    d. greater than +90 degrees

3. Limb Leads are V1 to V6 (True/False)

4. Chest leads are I, II, III, aVR, aVL and aVF (True/False)

5. A normal sinus rhythm has a P to QRS ratio of _

    a. 2:1

    b. 2:2

    c. 1:2

    d. 1:1

6. Anterior view is measured by leads _ and _.

7. Lateral view is monitored by leads _, _, _, and _.

8. The septum is monitored by leads _ and _.

9. The bottom of the heart is monitored by leads _, _, and _.

10. V4 lead is placed at the _ intercostal space.

    a. Third

    b. Fourth

    c. Fifth

    d. Sixth

Chapter 5

ECG Diagnosis

This is a list of ailments that can be diagnosed from ECG readings.

A

Accelerated Idioventricular Rhythm

Accelerated Idioventricular Rhythm occurs when the ectopic ventricular pacemaker works faster than the sinus node.

This kind of rhythm is most commonly observed during the reperfusion phase of acute STEMI (ST-Elevation Myocardial Infarction). It may be triggered by certain substances such as cocaine, anaesthetics, and beta-sympathomimetics (ex. Adrenaline and isoprenaline). Illnesses such as cardiomyopathy, myocarditis, congenital heart disease and electrolyte abnormalities may cause this rhythm. Return of spontaneous circulation (ROSC) after cardiac arrest or post thrombolysis (blood clot breakdown) may lead to this rhythm as well. However, athletic hearts may beat in this fashion but this is not usually a problem.

Accelerated Idioventricular Rhythm is a faster type of Idioventricular rhythm. It has a regular rhythm at 40-100 BPM. QRS is wide and deformed, measuring

120 ms or more. It has no P waves. In AV dissociation or third-degree heart block, accelerated idioventricular rhythm may contain P waves. It may include fusion and capture beats.

Treatment

AIVR is usually mild and does not need treatment most of the time. Like IVR, it is self-limiting, and normalizes when the sinus rate exceeds the ventricular rate. It is more important to treat the underlying causes, in order to improve prognosis. In some situations, however, AIVR may need to be inhibited, as it can worsen prognosis. This is seen in cases of loss of atrial-ventricular synchrony, relative rapid ventricular rate, and ventricular tachycardia or fibrillation. In these cases, atropine is used to increase the heart rate. Anti-arrhythmic agents are not used because this may lead to precipitous hemodynamic deterioration. Low cardiac output patients may be given atropine to increase AV conduction and sinus rate.

Accelerated Junctional Rhythm

This occurs in an AV junctional pacemaker that fires faster than the normal pacemaker (sinus node). The AV node experiences an increased automaticity, while the sinus node has decreased automaticity.

The classic cause of AJR is digoxin toxicity, but beta-agonists can also contribute to it. Heart ailments such as myocarditis and myocardial ischemia can sometimes provoke this rhythm. It is also an infrequent side-effect of cardiac surgery.

AJR has an above-average pace of 60-100 BPM; if beyond that, it is recognized as junctional tachycardia. If slower than 60 BPM, it is considered as junctional escape rhythm.

It is classified according to cause:

> » Automatic Junctional Rhythms, that are caused by increased automaticity in the cells of the AV node.

> » Re-entrant Junctional Rhythms, which are caused by a re-entrant loop in the AV node.

The QRS duration is narrow, usually measuring less than 120 ms except for cases of pre-existing bundle branch block or other conduction abnormalities. Ventricular rate is usually at 60-100 BPM. P waves may be retrograde and show up during, before, or after QRS complexes. They are usually inverted in the inferior leads (II, III, and aVF) and upright in aVr and V1.

If the ventricular rate is greater than the atrial rate, AV dissociation may be involved.

Rapid AJR (Automatic Junctional Tachycardia) is similar to re-entrant junctional tachycardias such as AVRT and AVNRT. The distinguishing factor of AJR is heart rate variability and rhythm irregularity. It does not usually respond to vagal stimulation – ventricular rate may temporarily slow down, but the sinus rhythm will not normalize.

Junctional tachycardia is around 115 BPM. P waves are retrograde and upright in V1 and aVr, while inverted in leads II, III, and aVF. The short PR interval measuring less than 120 ms implies a junctional focus.

AJR with aberrant conduction is similar to accelerated idioventricular rhythm. If there are fusion or capture beats, it is ventricular and not junctional.

Treatment

Management of accelerated junctional rhythm depends on the condition of the patient and the underlying cause of the abnormal rhythm. Asymptomatic patients, if the cause is normal physiological response, may not need treatment, especially if the rhythm is caused by a normal increase in vagal tone. However, patients in whom heart block is the cause must be treated. Those with AV blocks or sinus node dysfunction may benefit from having a pacemaker implanted. AJR caused by digoxin toxicity may be counteracted by medication such as Digibind and atropine.

For severe cases, radiofrequency ablation may be done to correct the rhythm.

Anterior STEMI

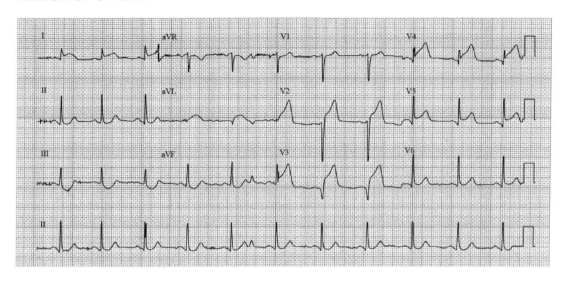

Figure 5. Acute anterior myocardial infarction, showing ST elevation in anterior leads (V1-6, I and aVL) and reciprocal ST depression in inferior leads.

Anterior STEMI (ST elevated myocardial infarction) is the blockage of the left anterior descending artery. This condition is considered the worst of all infarct cases.

Anterior STEMI is recognizable by ST segment elevation with Q waves in the precordial leads (V1 to V6) and/or high lateral leads (I and aVL). There is a reciprocal ST depression in the inferior leads (usually III and aVF).

The infarct patterns are based on the leads that display the most ST elevation:

- » Septal = V1 to V2
- » Anterior = V2 to V5
- » Anteroseptal = V1 to V4
- » Anterolateral = V3 to V6, I and aVL
- » Extensive anterior/anterolateral = V1 to V6, I and aVL

These are other things to look for:

» Left main coronary artery occlusion: general ST depression with ST elevation in aVR, that is greater or equal to V1

» Anterior-inferior STEMI caused by occlusion of left anterior descending artery: ST elevation in both precordial and inferior leads, because the blocked LAD wraps around the cardiac apex to supply the left ventricle's anterior and inferior walls

» Wellen's syndrome: deep T wave inversions in the precordial leads or biphasic T waves in V2 to V3, implying proximal LAD stenosis that may immediately lead to anterior infarction

» De Winter's T waves: upsloping ST depression, with symmetrical T waves in the precordial leads; a sign of acute LAD occlusion

Treatment

The mainstay of any MI is to establish reperfusion quickly, in order to salvage the myocardium. This may be done surgically or medically. Percutaneous coronary intervention, or coronary artery bypass grafting are the surgical techniques used. If this cannot be done immediately, medications that disintegrate clots (fibrinolytics) are used, such as streptokinase, along with blood thinners and platelet inhibitors. Oxygen is given to provide oxygenation to the blood in the absence of a properly functioning heart.

Arrhythmogenic Right Ventricular Dysplasia

Arrhythmogenic right ventricular dysplasia (enlargement or proliferation of abnormal cells) is a kind of cardiomyopathy (heart muscle disease) that does not involve blockages. It is also called as arrhythmogenic right ventricular cardiomyopathy (ARVC).

ARVC is an inherited disease of the right ventricular myocardium, where the normal muscle is replaced by fibrous fat. This is said to be the second most common reason for sudden cardiac death in young people below the age of 35. Those with a family history of sudden cardiac death may have ARVC.

ARVC is diagnosed with a combination of ECG and other imaging devices such as MRI, CT scans, and right ventricular contrast angiography.

The characteristics of ARVC are:

» Sustained ventricular tachycardia with LBBB morphology

» Ventricular ectopic beats

» Accompanied by syncope, palpitations, or cardiac arrest

» Can lead to right ventricular failure, severe biventricular failure, and/or dilated cardiomyopathy

The tell-tale sign of ARVC in an ECG is the Epsilon wave but it is only seen in around 1/3 of patients. Almost all, however have prolonged S-wave upstrokes of 55 ms in V1 to V3, as well as T wave inversions in V1 to V3. There is localized widening of the QRS complexes, measuring 110 ms in V1 to V3. Ventricular tachycardia with LBBB morphology comes in paroxysms.

Treatment

ARVC is treated by anti-arrhythmic medication such as sotalol, amiodarone, or conventional beta-blockers such as metoprolol. Those with urgent symptoms can benefit from an implantable cardioverter-defibrillator (ICD) which is very effective in preventing sudden cardiac death. Patients with persistent ARVC can be given radiofrequency ablation of the conduction pathways.

If this progresses to heart failure, ACE inhibitors, diuretics, and anti-coagulants are given. Heart transplant may also be done for extensive damage which cannot be treated with pharmacological intervention.

Atrial Flutter

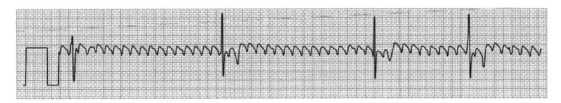

Figure 6. Atrial flutter showing 'sawtooth' or 'picket-fence' appearance.

Atrial flutter is a form of supraventricular tachycardia, that is triggered by a re-entry circuit in the right atrium.

The atrial rate is dependent on the atrium size, and is usually 250-350 BPM, while ventricular rate is determined by the AV conduction ratio or the degree of the AV block, and is often around 125-175 BPM.

The AV ratio is often 2:1, but medications or heart disease can result into lower rates.

1:1 conduction may be caused by sympathetic stimulation, or an accessory pathway, such as when AV-nodal blocking agents were given to a WPW patient. It is also linked to severe hemodynamic instability and may progress to ventricular fibrillation.

F waves manifest in a saw-tooth pattern. The QRS rate is often regular and complexes appear at some multiple of the P-P interval. There may be 2 F waves for every QRS complex. The ventricular response may have 3:1 or higher rates. It may also be irregular.

Treatment

The first choice of treatment for atrial flutter is radiofrequency ablation, which is believed to be superior to medical therapy because it has a decreased risk of associated complications. Synchronized electrical cardioversion is done for flutters of short duration (< 48 hours). Patient must be immediately started on anticoagulation therapy, to prevent thromboembolic complications. In cases where ablation is not feasible, anti-arrhythmic agents, such as dofetilide, or ibutilide are used. If the heart function is normal, beta-adrenergic blockers or calcium channel blockers are given concurrently.

Atrial Fibrillation

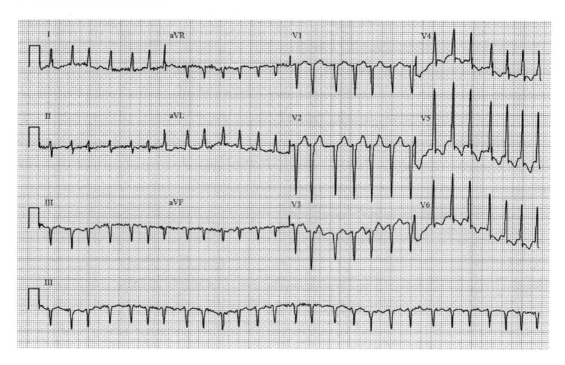

Figure 7. Atrial fibrillation depicting typical irregularly irregular ventricular rhythm.

Atrial fibrillation happens when atrial pacemaker cells fire randomly. This is the most common form of sustained arrhythmia. It is caused by several factors: ischemic or valvular heart disease, pericardial disease, dilated or hypertrophic cardiomyopathies, hypertension, pulmonary embolus, acute infections, thyrotoxicosis, phaeochromocytoma, electrolyte imbalances (hypomagnesaemia, hypokalemia), acid-base imbalance, and certain drugs.

Atrial fibrillation has an irregularly irregular pattern with a ventricular rate of about 110-160 BPM in general. It is categorized as a "rapid ventricular response" if it is over 100 BPM and "slow" if it is below 60 BPM. Slow AF is caused by sinus mode dysfunction, hypothermia, digoxin toxicity, and some medications.

There are no P waves, and the QRS complexes are usually less than 120 ms, unless there is an accessory pathway, bundle branch block, or other conduction problem. There is no set P:QRS ratio or PR interval.

This may contain fibrillatory waves that may sometimes resemble P waves.

Atrial Fibrillation in WPW

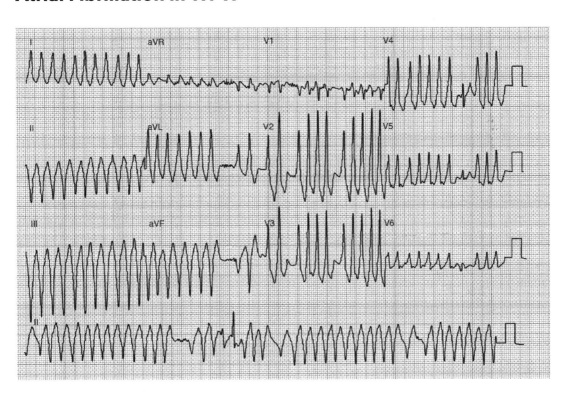

Figure 8. Wolf-Parkinson-White syndrome with atrial fibrillation and an irregularly irregular, wide complex tachycardia.

Wolff-Parkinson-White syndrome is a congenital condition in which there are abnormal conductive pathways between the atria and ventricles. 1/5 of people with WPW will tend to have atrial fibrillation because the accessory pathway directs conduction to the ventricles without passing the AV node. Rhythm is irregular, and rates exceed 200 BPM. QRS complexes are wide and erratic because of abnormal ventricular depolarization. Axis remains stable though, unlike in Polymorphic VT.

Treatment

Treatment in a hemodynamically stable individual include either medical methods, such as ibutilide or procainamide, or DC cardioversion. In a hemodynamically unstable one, urgent synchronized DC cardioversion is recommended. Anticoagulants such as warfarin or heparin should be used to prevent stroke in almost all patients suffering from AF, except those who are at a higher risk of bleeding.

Cryoablation or radiofrequency ablation is the recommended surgical mode of treatment in younger patients where rhythm cannot be controlled by pharmacological intervention or cardioversion.

AF should not be treated with AV nodal blocking drugs (beta-blockers, calcium channel blockers, adenosine) because these may increase the conduction through the accessory pathway, which will speed up ventricular rate and degenerate to VF or VT.

In Wolff-Parkinson-White syndrome, therapy is aimed at removing the accessory pathway, which is usually achieved by radiofrequency ablation of that pathway. Anti-arrhythmic drugs, as described above, can also be used to slow conduction.

Atrial Ectopic Beat/Atrial Premature Beat

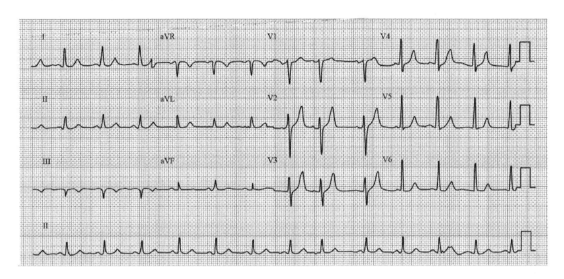

Figure 9. Atrial Premature Beat (APB) characterized by an abnormal P wave and a small compensatory pause.

In this, the ECG shows an abnormal P wave leading the ectopic beat and a small compensatory pause following it. This is also known by other terms, such as atrial premature depolarizations, Premature Atrial Contraction (PAC). This condition does not usually require treatment, however, in those that have other heart problems, a PAC may lead to re-entrant tachydysrhythmia.

All these terms that are defined as a premature beat originate from an ectopic focus in the atria.

PAC happens when another pacemaker cell in the atria fires faster than the SA node. This causes the complex to arrive earlier than normal. The premature beat resets the SA node, thus the rhythm is disturbed.

The rhythm is irregular. The P wave exists but is abnormal.

P: QRS ratio is 1:1 but the PR interval varies. QRS is normal. There may sometimes be grouping but there are no dropped beats.

PAC may be provoked by diverse things: excess caffeine intake, anxiety, beta-agonists, sympathomimetics, digoxin toxicity, myocardial ischemia, hypokalemia, or hypomagnesaemia.

Treatment

Since most of these premature beats are benign, they do not need treatment. Sometimes, PAC may require treatment, especially if it is associated with an underlying disease. In these cases, either beta blockers or anti-arrhythmic agents may be prescribed.

Atrial Tachycardia

Atrial tachycardia is also known as ectopic atrial tachycardia, paroxysmal atrial tachycardia (PAT), unifocal atrial tachycardia, and multifocal atrial tachycardia.

It is a fast beat originating from the atria but outside the sinus node.

This is commonly due to one ectopic focus but there can also be several foci. Causes may be idiopathic, or due to digoxin toxicity, catecholamine excess, atrial scarring, or congenital defects.

As with tachycardia in general, atrial tachycardia has an atrial rate of greater than 100 BPM. Because the P wave is ectopic, it looks different from normal. Atrial tachycardia has at least 3 consecutive ectopic P waves that are identical. The inferior leads (II, III, aVF) show an inverted P-wave axis. The QRS complexes are often normal.

Atrial tachycardia can be distinguished from atrial flutter because the former has an isoelectric baseline, while the latter does not.

Treatment

The primary goal during an episode of atrial tachycardia should be rate control by using AV nodal blocking drugs. Many episodes of atrial tachycardia can terminate if the cause is addressed. If it persists, however, the episode may be teminated by the use of agents that block the AV node (beta blockers and calcium channel blockers). Carotid sinus massages or Valsalva's manoeuvres may also be performed to correct atrial tachycardia. If the patient is unstable, such as a child with complex congenital heart disease, urgent synchronized electrical cardioversion is given.

Surgical ablation should be performed in patients with complex congenital heart disease.

AV block: 1ˢᵗ degree / First-Degree Heart Block

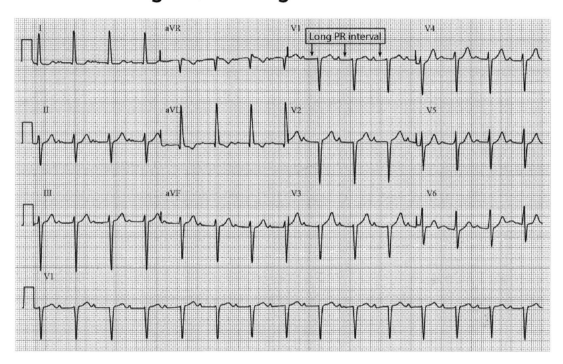

Figure 10. AV node block showing long PR interval

This happens when the AV node experiences a prolonged block because of vagal stimulation, medication (eg. AV nodal blocking drugs), and health conditions such as inferior MI, myocarditis, and electrolyte imbalances, or as a side-effect of mitral valve surgery. Athletes may also experience this. This does not require treatment and does not cause hemodynamic problems.

The PR interval is greater than 200 milliseconds. If greater than 300 ms, it is considered as a marked first degree block.

The rhythm is regular. The P wave is normal and has a 1:1 ratio to the QRS. The QRS width is likewise normal, and there are no dropped beats or groupings.

Treatment

The treatment depends on the underlying cause of the block. If asymptomatic, usually no treatment is required. However, if the block is marked (PR interval> 300 ms), cardiac pacemakers may be beneficial. Pharmacological therapy may also be used, including atropine and isoproternerol. Use of AV node blocking agents must be avoided, and discontinued. Any electrolyte imbalances must be identified and corrected. Hospitalization may be required in first-degree heart block patients presenting with associated myocardial infarction.

AV block: 2nd degree, Mobitz 1 (Wenckebach)

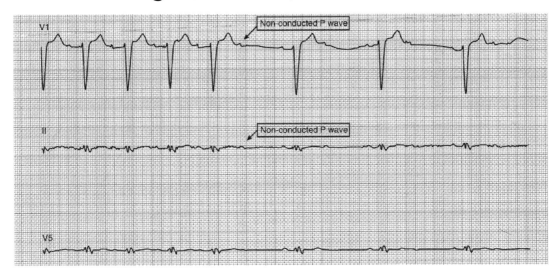

Figure 11. 2 to 1 AV block where every other P wave is conducted; cannot be labeled as a Mobitz type I or II pattern

A diseased AV node, with a prolonged refractory period causes this condition. The conduction block is reversible, however. This is usually benign; those without symptoms don't need treatment while those who do often get better with atropine.

Causes of Mobitz I are increased vagal tone, myocarditis, inferior MI, post cardiac surgery (example repair of mitral valve or Tetralogy of Fallot), and some drugs.

The PR interval lengthens between beats until a beat is dropped, then the cycle restarts. The P-P interval is relatively consistent, but the R-R interval shortens with every beat.

The rhythm is regularly irregular. The P wave is present, but the P:QRS ratio varies (2:1, 5:4, 4:3, etc.) such as in Wenkebach.

The PR interval is variable and is at its longest before a dropped beat and shortest after it. The QRS width is normal. Grouping may exist and may be variable. There are dropped beats.

Treatment

This does not require specific therapy if the patient is asymptomatic. The cause of the AV block is identified and managed. Drugs such as digoxin, beta blockers, and calcium channel blockers may be discontinued, or the dose may be reduced. Atropine, isoproterenol, and transcutaneous pacing may be given for symptomatic cases, until the arrhythmia is gone.

AV block: 2nd degree, Mobitz II / Mobitz II Second-Degree Heart Block

This is more commonly caused by conduction failure of the His-Purkinje system because of structural damage (ex. Fibrosis, infarction, necrosis). This is more serious than Mobitz I because it can lead to complete heart block.

Those with LBBB or bifascicular block tend to have Mobitz II. There are several causes: idiopathic fibrosis, anterior MI, infiltrative myocardial disease, autoimmune, cardiac surgery, hyperkalemia, and drug toxicity.

There are grouped beats with a beat dropped between groupings. The PR interval is the same for all of the conducted beats.

Like Mobitz I, the rhythm is also regularly irregular. There are P waves that have variable P:QRS ratios.

PR interval is normal.

QRS may be wide when the conduction block occurs distal to the His Bundle, and narrow when it's in the His Bundle.

Groupings are present and may vary. Dropped beats are observable.

Treatment

As with Mobitz 1 block, agents that can block AV node must be avoided or reduced. Transcutaneous cardiac pacing is the treatment of choice and must be done as soon as possible. Dopamine, epinephrine, or a combination of both may be given through I.V. infusion.

For serious cases, a permanent pacemaker may be necessary.

AV block: 3rd degree (complete heart block) / Third-Degree Heart Block

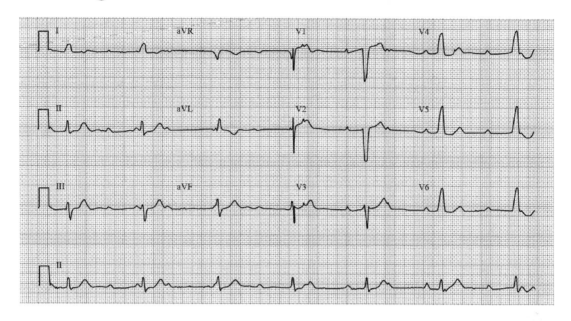

Figure 12. Complete Heart Block showing no correlation between P waves and QRS complexes

This is a total block of the AV node, where the atria and ventricles are firing on their own. The sinus rhythm may be normal, or faster or slower than expected. The escape beat can be junctional or ventricular.

Sinus rhythm and escape rhythm have their own rates, and are dissociated from each other. Rhythm is regular but P and QRS rate are dissimilar. P waves are there but P:QRS ratio is variable. PR interval is variable and has no discernible pattern. QRS width may be wide or normal. There are no dropped beats or grouping.

Remember: when there are the same number of P waves and QRS complexes, but they are dissociated, it is AV dissociation and not third-degree heart block.

Treatment

As with the previous heart blocks, transcutaneous pacing is the treatment of choice. Any causative medications must be withdrawn, and I.V. infusion of epinephrine and/or dopamine may be given. Installation of a permanent pacemaker or an implantable cardioverter defibrillator (ICD) may also be considered in patients with complete heart block. Atropine is indicated when the patient is hemodynamically unstable, however, atropine is contraindicated when there are wide-complex ventricular escape beats.

AVNRT (AV-nodal re-entry tachycardia) / Supraventricular Tachycardia (SVT)

AVNRT and SVT are one and the same, however they can be used to describe any tachydysrhythmia (fast abnormal beat) originating above the His Bundle.

AVNRT/SVT is the most common cause of palpitations among those with normally structured hearts. It is provoked by caffeine, physical exertion, alcohol, beta-agonists, or sympathomimetics. This is generally non-fatal, even among those with heart disease.

This is produced by the AV node or atria, and usually results into tachycardia (140-280 BPM) with narrow complexes (less than 120 ms), unless there are other problems present. P waves may be visible and display inversion (retrograde conduction) in leads II, III, and aVF, positioned after the QRS complex, or at rare times, before it. It can also be hidden in the QRS complex.

SVTs are categorized according to origin and regularity:

Atrial

» Regular rhythm: Atrial flutter, Atrial tachycardia, Sinus tachycardia, Sinus node re-entrant tachycardia, Inappropriate sinus tachycardia

» Irregular rhythm: Atrial flutter with variable block, Atrial fibrillation, Multifocal atrial tachycardia

Atrioventricular

> » AV nodal re-entry tachycardia (AVNRT)
> » Atrioventricular re-entry tachycardia (AVRT)
> » Automatic junctional tachycardia

Treatment

The treatment of AVNRT depends on the patients' cardiac history and previous ECGs. AVNRT management includes vagal manoeuvres, such as carotid sinus massage and Valsalva manuover, preferably with the patient in Trendelenberg position. However, these are contraindicated if hypotension is present. Pharmacological therapy may be used to terminate an attack by slowing down conduction through the AV node, including medication, such as adenosine. Recurrence is avoided by use of calcium-channel blockers, beta-blockers, and amiodarone. Asthmatic patients should be closely monitored as adenosine and beta-blockers can cause congestion of the airways. If the patient does not respond to pharmacotherapy, or has hemodynamic compromise, DC synchronized cardioversion may be applied. Those who do not respond to regular treatment may be given catheter ablation.

AVRT (Atrioventricular Re-Entry Tachycardia)

This is a tachyarrhythmia caused by a re-entry circuit in the normal conduction system, or a direct conduction from the atria to ventricles through an accessory pathway, as is seen in Wolff-Parkinson_white syndrome.

This is often provoked by premature atrial or ventricular beats.

Treatment

Treatment is similar to AVNRT. Vagal manoeuvres may be attempted before starting drug treatments, but should not be done if the patient has low blood pressure. Direct current synchronized cardioversion may terminate the attack if the patient is hemodynamically compromised or if the drug treatment does not work. Competitive atrial or ventricular pacing may be used if cardioversion is not permitted.

B

Benign Early Repolarization / High Take Off / J-Point Elevation

Benign early repolarization is seen among healthy individuals who are less than 50 years old. Although benign, this resembles acute MI or pericarditis.

BER is recognizable by widespread concave elevation of the ST segments, especially in the mid to left precordial leads (V2 to V5). The J-points have notches. The T-waves are prominent and slightly asymmetrical and points at the same direction as the QRS complexes.

The ST elevation is usually less than ¼ of the height of the T wave in V6. It is generally less than 2 mm in the precordial leads and less than 0.5 mm in the limb leads.

Treatment

Asymptomatic patients may not need to be treated, as the name indicates that the condition is benign. Symptoms that may manifest are given remedies. If the patients has experienced ventricular fibrillation, or sudden cardiac arrest, an implantable cardioverter defibrillator may be placed.

Beta-Blocker Toxicity

This rhythm is caused by excessive intake of beta-blockers such as atenolol, propranolol, metoprolol, and sotalol and some cardioselective calcium-channel blockers like diltiazem and verapamil.

The ECG shows bradycardia (sinus, ventricular, and/or junctional), and/or 1st/2nd/3rd degree AV block.

Treatment

The goal of treatment is to increase the cardiac output, by increasing the heart rate and improving myocardial contractility. Hypotension, bradycardia, and seizures should be prepared for. Charcoal (not Ipecac syrup) may be indicated to help flush out the substance via gastric decontamination.

If the patient is hypotensive, 20ml/kg of isotonic intravenous fluids may be given while he/she is in the Trendelenburg position.

The following protocol is recommended if the patient does not respond to above mentioned measures.

- » Glucagon
- » High-dose insulin
- » Inotropes and chronotropes
- » Benzodiapenes (for seizures)
- » Hemodialysis
- » Extracorporeal membrane oxygenation
- » Cardiac pacing and/or resuscitations

Bidirectional VT

This is a rare type of ventricular dysrhythmia that shows beat-to-beat alternation along the frontal QRS axis. This can signify an alternating left and right bundle-branch lock.

Bidirectional VT is most commonly observed in cases of severe digoxin toxicity, but also among those with herbal aconite poisoning. Individuals with familial catecholaminergic polymorphic ventricular tachycardia (CPVT) also have this rhythm.

Treatment

If bidirectional VT is caused by digoxin, Digibind is used (2 – 20 ampoules, depending on severity). If caused by AV block, atropine 0.6 mg bolus is given intravenously. Intravenous lignocaine can also treat the arrhythmia. Hyperkalemia is counteracted by insulin, dextrose, and sodium bicarbonate, but not with calcium given intravenously.

Bidirectional VT may cause cardiac arrest; patients may need continuous CPR until Digibind becomes available. DC cardioversion is ineffective for this condition.

Catecolaminergic Polymorphic Ventricular Tachycardia is treated by beta-blockers, electrical cardioversion or defibrillation, and an implantable cardioverter-defibrillator.

Bifascicular Block

A bifascicular block is RBBB (right bundle branch block), coinciding with LPFB (Left Posterior Fascicular Block) or LAFB (Left Anterior Fascicular Block). This implies an extensive conducting system disorder, but rarely progresses to complete heart block. The conduction arriving at the ventricles is done through the remaining fascicle.

The main causes of this kind of block are ischemic heart disease, hypertension, anterior MI, aortic stenosis, congenital heart disease, degenerative disease of the conductive system, and hyperkalemia.

The ECG displays RBBB traits and a deviation to the left or right axis.

Treatment

Management depends on the cause of the bifascicular block. The underlying cause must be analyzed and treated appropriately. Those with no symptoms do not usually need treatment; those who do (e.g. repeated episodes of syncope) may benefit from a pacemaker, which will regularize the rhythm. Patients with renal disease or structural heart disease also have higher risk of progressing to trifascicular block. Hence, this group requires continuous monitoring, and pacemaker insertion may also be considered in these patients.

Biventricular Enlargement

This is the hypertrophy or enlargement of both ventricles.

The main ECG features of this condition are a combination of LVH and RVH indicators; however, it may be hard to detect since LVH and RVH often negate each other. A more obvious sign is the Katz Wachtel phenomenon, where large biphasic QRS complexes are witnessed in V2 to V5.

In case of confirmed LVH, additional signs to look out for to confirm Biventricular Enlargement are right axis deviation, right atrial enlargement (as seen in other imaging studies), deep S waves in V5 to V6, and tall biphasic QRS complexes in several leads.

In case of confirmed RVH, indicators for biventricular enlargement are QRS complexes that are greater than 50 mm, tall R waves and deep S waves in leads V2 to V5.

Treatment

Treatment focuses on addressing the cause. In cases of systemic hypertension, medication that lowers blood pressure may help with normalizing the size of the ventricles. These include ACE inhibitors, ARBs, beta/calcium channel blockers, and diuretics. Digoxin may be administered to enhance the pumping function of the heart. If the enlargement is caused by stenosis, surgery may be done to repair or replace the faulty valve. Patients with coronary artery disease need to undergo removal of blockages, to improve blood flow by performing coronary bypass surgery. Heart transplant is the last option if all of the above treatment modes fail to respond.

Biatrial Enlargement

This is enlargement of both atria that may be caused by pulmonary hypertension, hypertension, congenital heart disease, aortic or tricuspid stenosis, hypertrophic cardiomyopathy, mitral incompetence, mitral/aortic valve disease, or chronic lung disease.

Biatrial enlargement is diagnosed when there are indicators of both left and right atrial hypertrophy on the ECG.

In Lead II, the bifid P wave is equal to or greater than 2.5 mm and equal to or greater than 120 ms.

In V1, biphasic P waves has an initial positive deflection measuring 1.5 mm or greater and has a terminal negative deflection 1mm deep or greater and 40 ms or greater in duration.

Combination criteria includes P wave positive deflection 1.5 mm and above in leads V1 or V2 and notched P waves greater than 120 ms in limb leads and V5 or V6.

Treatment

As with biventricular enlargement, the cause of the condition is addressed. Enlarged atria may be treated by controlling hypertension through ACE inhibitors, beta blockers, and diuretics. Anticoagulants and anti-arrhythmics should also be administered along with these medications. Potassium supplements may be given to correct heart conduction problems. Implantable cardioverter-defibrillator (ICD) may be recommended for patients at risk of developing serious arrhythmias. Surgery is required for correcting structural abnormalities, such as faulty valves, which would require replacement.

Brugada Syndrome

Brugada syndrome is named after the Brugada brothers who first described the condition.

This is linked to Sudden Unexplained Nocturnal Death Syndrome (SUNDS).

It is due to a genetic mutation in the cardiac sodium channel, also known as sodium channelopathy.

Conditions accompanying it are fever, hypothermia, ischemia, hypokalemia, drugs (pharmaceutical and recreational), and post DC cardioversion.

This condition is diagnosed by the Brugada sign, an ST segment elevation of greater than 2 mm in more than 1 lead of V1 to V3 and followed by a negative T wave.

To confirm this diagnosis, the following criteria must be met:

- » Presence of polymorphic ventricular tachycardia or ventricular fibrillation.
- » Inducible VTs with electrical stimulation
- » Family history of sudden cardiac death while aged below 45 years old
- » Family members also have coved ECGs
- » Syncope (loss of consciousness)
- » Difficulty in breathing during sleeping

Treatment

The best way to treat Brugada syndrome is with the implantation of a cardioverter-defibrillator (ICD). Patients with Brugada syndrome, who have survived cardiac arrest, are candidates for ICD implantation, while asymptomatic patients do not require it, but must be monitored closely. Family history of sudden cardiac death is another reason to consider ICD implantation.

No medications have been proved to be effective in preventing sudden death in patients with Brugada syndrome.

C

Calcium-channel blocker toxicity

This is a lethal condition that causes the heart to collapse, but the patient can be saved by providing thorough treatment and circulatory support.

The most toxic overdoses come from diltiazem and verapamil. Since these two and other channel blockers like them prevent the influx of calcium to the heart cells, too much of them can interfere with the heartbeat and dilate the blood vessels.

Symptoms are chest pains, palpitations, difficulty breathing, vomiting, seizures, sweating, dizziness, and fainting. Blood pressure is low and heart rate is slow.

In the ECG, this manifests as bradycardia, AV block, bundle branch block, and ST segment and T wave abnormalities.

Treatment

Managing this condition involves life support protocol; manage the airway, breathing and circulation of the patient, while correcting electrolyte and acid-base imbalances. Crystalloid fluid boluses are given to flush out the drug. Bradycardia is treated with atropine. Activated charcoal given orally may help absorb and flush out the toxic substance if taken within an hour of poisoning. Ipecac syrup is strongly contraindicated as it may increase the risk of seizures.

Specific medications used are calcium to overcome the channel blockade, , lipid emulsion therapy agents, high-dose insulin and glucagon to promote calcium entry into cells, and vasopressors.

Carbamazepine Cardiotoxicity

Carbamazepine overdose (greater than 50 mg/kg) creates this condition because of fast sodium channel blockade.

Symptoms of carbamazepine overdose or toxicity includes hallucinations, blurred eyesight, nausea, vomiting, seizures, tremors, loss of control of body movements (ataxia) and rapid unintentional movement of eyes (nystagmus). Urine output is reduced because of the alteration of sodium levels in the blood.

Heart rate is fast and blood pressure is dangerously low. This causes QRS widening or sometimes 1st degree AV block. There may be a small secondary R wave in the lead aVR.

Treatment

As with most poisoning cases, charcoal may be given to remove the carbamazepine from the body, for as long as he/she is still conscious and the airway is clear. Do not induce vomiting, in order to prevent CNS depression and seizures. In case seizure results, diazepam or other benzodiapenes will help to control them.

IV fluids may be administered, especially if the patient is hypotensive. Whole-bowel irrigation should be performed. The guidelines recommend 1.5-2 litres/hour of polyethylene glycol lavage solution for adults, whereas, children should be treated with 0.5 litres/hour. If the QRS is wider than 100 ms, give sodium bicarbonate to counter sodium channel blockade.

Cardiomyopathy, Dilated

This is a fatal heart disease involving dilatation of the ventricles, and overall heart dysfunction. It has two common types: ischemic, following a massive anterior MI, and non-ischemic/genetic. Others causes include viral myocarditis, toxins, autoimmune disease, pregnancy, and alcoholism.

Dilated cardiomyopathy has no specific indicator, unlike Brugada syndrome but the ECG looks abnormal in general. It shares common signs with hypertrophy (atrial, biatrial, ventricular, biventricular). There are intraventricular delays because of cardiac dilatation.

QRS complexes have reduced voltage in the limb leads because of myocardial fibrosis. Abnormal Q waves are observed in V1 to V4, and may resemble an MI pattern.

Treatment

Dilated cardiomyopathy is treated similar to chronic heart failure. This is treated with antihypertensives, including vasodilators, diuretics, cardiac glycosides, ACE inhibitors, and beta-blockers. Anti-coagulants are given to thin blood and prevent clots. If arrhythmias are present, anti-arrhythmic drugs are given. Surgical options include left ventricular assist devices, implantable cardioverter-defibrillators, biventricular pacing, ventricular restoration surgery, and heart transplants.

Cardiomyopathy, Hypertrophic

Hypertrophic cardiomyopathy (HCM) was previously called as hypertrophic obstructive cardiomyopathy (HOCM) and idiopathic hypertrophic subaortic stenosis (IHSS).

This is one of the most prevalent inherited disorders of the heart, and is the leading cause of mortality in athletes.

This manifests as a dynamic obstruction of the left ventricular outflow tract (LVOT). The left ventricle's diastole is abnormal, because of its inability to relax and fill up sufficiently. The intramural coronary arteries have thick walls and narrowed passageways. There is a disorganized transmission of electrical impulses, which can lead to arrhythmia.

The effects of this condition are syncope, chest pain, palpitations, and pulmonary congestion. It can sometimes lead to cardiac death.

The ECG shows signs of left atrial hypertrophy, left ventricular hypertrophy (abnormal T waves and ST segments), deep and narrow Q waves in the inferior and lateral leads, huge T wave inversions in the precordial leads, signs of WPW (delta waves and short PR), and other dysrhythmias.

Treatment

This is treated by medication (beta blockers, calcium channel blockers, anti-arrhythmic agents, blood thinners). Surgery may be done to remove tissue overgrowth, for example, septal myectomy. Septal ablation involves destroying the thickened heart muscle, by injecting alcohol through a catheter. For life-threatening conditions, an implantable cardioverter-defibrillator is implanted.

Cardiomyopathy, Restrictive

Restrictive cardiomyopathy occurs during advanced myocardial infiltrative disease.

Ventricular arrhythmias and atrial fibrillation tend to accompany this condition.

There are low-voltage QRS complexes and unusual Q waves.

T waves and ST segments are abnormal.

Indicators of bundle branch blocks are present. AV block may also be involved, and in the case of sarcoidosis, may manifest as a 3rd degree AV block.

ECG may show atrial and ventricular dysrhythmias

Treatment

The treatment for restrictive cardiomyopathy is targeted to its particular causes. Symptomatic treatment can be given to reduce congestion, lower filling pressure, and prevent embolism. This is achieved by use of vasodilators, diuretics, and ACE inhibitors. If not contraindicated, anti-coagulants may also help in preventing thromboembolism. Permanent pacing, LVAD therapy, and heart transplantation may be done on certain patients, who do not respond to pharmacotherapy.

Chronic Obstructive Pulmonary Disease (COPD)

COPD affects the heart rhythm, and causes ECG changes. When the lungs over expand, the heart becomes compressed and the diaphragm lowers, causing the heart to become longer and to be vertically oriented. It can rotate clockwise, with the right ventricle moving slightly forwards and left ventricle moving slightly backwards.

Because of the new position and an excess of air surrounding the heart, the electrical signals may become weakened. The QRS complexes will show this and have reduced amplitude.

Other ECG traits are as follows:

The P wave axis shifts to the right, with P waves prominent among the inferior leads and inverted or flat in leads I and aVL.

The QRS wave axis also shifts to the right. QRS voltages are low especially in the left precordial leads (V4 to V6).

Atrial depolarization is amplified, resulting to ST and PR segments that dip below the baseline.

The R waves may be totally gone in leads V1 to V3.

COPD effects may also include signs seen in RBBB, and multifocal atrial tachycardia.

Treatment

The primary goal of treatment should be to optimize the lung function, reduce severity of symptoms, and prevent recurrence. The cause/s of the COPD is treated. Medications that reduce shortness of breath, control coughing fits, and prevent the recurrence of the condition are used. Beta-2 agonists and anticholinergic drugs are used to provide vasodilatation. Inflammation is managed by using oral or inhaled steroids. If infection sets in, doxycycline is preferred. Long-term antibiotics such as erythromycin may be recommended in patients with two or more than two episodes of COPD per year. Mucolytic agents such as n-acetyl cysteine can be used to reduce secretions. Oxygen is given to assist with the patient's breathing. Refractory cases might require lung transplantation.

D

De Winter's T waves

This rhythm gets its name from de Winter and Wellens, who observed it among patients with acute LAD blockages. It is now known that this ECG pattern can predict the condition quite accurately.

This is an anterior STEMI equivalent, but without an apparent elevation of the ST segments.

The most noticeable features are peaked and symmetrical T waves and depressed ST segments in the precordial leads. The ST depression measures greater than 1 mm at the J-point, and 0.5 – 1 mm in aVR. There is no ST elevation in the precordial leads.

Treatment

When a patient has De Winter's T waves, it means that he/she is experiencing STEMI.. Oxygen, morphine, nitroglycerin and aspirin are given primarily, as necessary. Fibrinolytic therapy is started to lyse the blood clot. PCI or CABG must be done to restablish reperfusion.

Dextrocardia

This is a rare condition where the heart's apex is at the right side of the body (instead of the normal left).

The ECG reflects a right axis deviation with positive QRS complexes and upright P and T waves in the lead aVR.

In Lead I, the complexes are all inverted.

S waves are dominant in the chest leads, and R wave progression is noticeably absent.

Take note that the reversal of the right and left electrodes may cause this pattern. Check whether the leads are placed correctly.

Treatment

Dextrocardia may cause complications such as frequent infections, and intestinal obstructions. These are treated by antibiotics and surgery.

Heart abnormalities are sometimes associated with holes in the septum, which can be remedied by surgical correction and pacemakers.

Digoxin effect

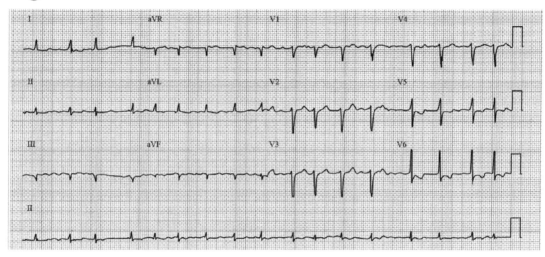

Figure 13. Digoxin effect showing characteristic 'reverse tick' appearance (down sloping ST depression, visible here in leads V5 and V6), dysrhythmias, and shortened QT interval.

Digoxin is a cardiac stimulant. It affects ECG readings.

Digoxin shortens the refractory period of the atrium and ventricles, and increases the vagal effects in the SA node.

It creates ST depressions that appear to sag, as well as shortened QT intervals. It makes the T waves become inverted, flat, or biphasic.

Other indicators of digoxin effect are big U waves, peaked terminal parts of T waves, slight PR interval prolongation of up to 240 ms, and J point depression mainly in leads with tall R waves.

Treatment

Digoxin effect is not treated unless it produces unpleasant symptoms (see the following section).

Digoxin Toxicity

Digoxin toxicity results when too much digoxin is taken, and the body reacts adversely.

Symptoms include nausea, vomiting, diarrhoea, blurred and abnormal vision, palpitations, difficulty breathing, confusion, dizziness, and fainting.

Several types of dysrhythmias may result because of increased automaticity and decreased AV conduction.

The classic sign of digoxin toxicity is a mixture of supraventricular tachycardia and slow ventricular response.

There may be frequent PVC and ventricular bigeminy or trigeminy. Sinus rhythm may be slow and there may be slow AF.

AV blocks may exist.

Ventricular tachycardia may also be there especially polymorphic and bidirectional VT.

Treatment

For acute overdose, activated charcoal is given to help eliminate the digoxin. Digoxin Immune Fab is the most effective medication for this kind of toxicity. Electrolyte imbalances are corrected, while dysrhythmias are treated with medication such as beta-blockers, lidocaine, phenytoin, and atropine.

Calcium channel blockers are contraindicated because they can enhance digoxin levels. Magnesium sulfate can help stop dysrhythmias but it is prohibited among those with AV block, bradycardia, or renal failure. Cardioversion should be attempted cautiously because this can lead to ventricular fibrillation and asystole.

E

Ectopic Atrial Tachycardia

This condition takes place when the ectopic atrial focus fires faster than the sinus rate. The P waves and PR intervals are dissimilar, because the rhythm is created by a pacemaker other than the normal SA node. This usually occurs only briefly. Because of the faster rate, some ST and T wave abnormalities may appear temporarily.

The rate is at 100-180 BPM but has a regular rhythm. The P wave's ectopic focus has a different form. The P:QRS ratio is 1:1. In the PR interval, the ectopic focus has a different interval. The QRS width may be normal or not. There are no groupings or dropped beats.

Treatment

Patients not having cardiac failure may be given intravenous class Ia and Ic anti-arrhythmics, such as quinidine or propafenone. Those with abnormal ventricular function are prescribed intravenous amiodarone. Class III anti-arrhythmic drugs do not always correct ectopic atrial tachycardia, but they help with maintaining normal sinus rhythm after conversion. Digoxin and beta-blockers may also be recommended to control heart rate. Radiofrequency ablation is also curative for ectopic atrial tachycardia.

Electrical Alternans

This is a condition caused by the heart swinging to and fro, in a huge pericardium filled with fluid. This creates normally conducted QRS complexes that have alternate heights.

Treatment

The primary goal is to treat the underlying cause. Long QT syndrome should be treated by withholding any causative drugs and correcting metabolic disturbances. Electrical alternans may not require surgery, but if it originates from pulmonary emboli, pulmonary embolectomy is done. Left-sided cervicothoracic sympathetic gangliectomy may be necessary for those with congenital long QT syndrome who do not respond to drug therapy. Pericardectomy is indicated for recurrent pericardial effusions.

F

Fascicular VT

This is the most prevalent idiopathic ventricular tachycardia. Healthy people may experience this when stressed, while exercising, after taking beta-agonists, or sometimes even during rest

The first treatment done is usually administering of Verapamil.

ECG signs are:

>> RBBB indicators with a left axis deviation (posterior fascicular VT)

>> RBBB indicators with a right axis deviation (anterior fascicular VT)

>> RBBB that may resemble LBBB, with narrow QRS complexes and normal axis arising from upper septum region (upper septal fascicular VT)

Treatment

Verapamil is fascicular VT's first line of treatment for stable patients with moderate symptoms, given at a dose of 120-480 mg/day. If the patient has severe symptoms, or is intolerant or resistant to anti-arrhythmias, catheter ablation should be performed. For emergency cases, electrical cardioversion is done.

H

High take-off

(See Benign Early Repolarization)

Hypercalcemia

Hypercalcemia is an excess of calcium in the blood. Because calcium is involved with the action potential of cells, an excess of it will result in conduction abnormalities of the heart.

Causes of hypercalcemia are:

- » Hyperparathyroidism
- » Sarcoidosis
- » Paraneoplastic syndromes
- » Bony metastases
- » Milk-alkali syndrome
- » Excess vitamin D

This condition appears in the ECG as strange-looking QRS complexes, extremely short QT intervals, and J waves (notches in the terminal QRS complex especially in V1)

Treatment

Fluid volume loss associated with hypercalcemia is treated with isotonic sodium chloride solution. When the volume has normalized, loop diuretics are given to block sodium and calcium reabsorption. Bisphosphonates may be used to prevent osteoclastic activity.

If the hypercalcemia is caused by hyperparathyroidism, surgical intervention may be necessary to remove the parathyroid gland.

Hyperkalemia

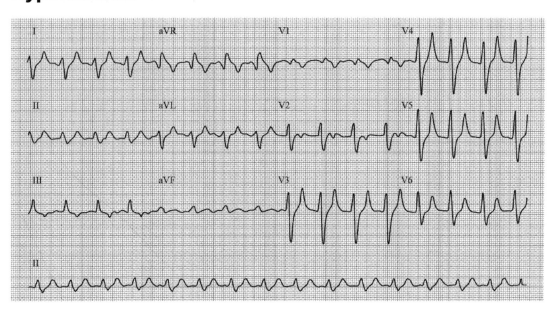

Figure 14. Hyperkalemia is characterized by tall and tented T waves, small or absent P waves and ST segments, wide QRS, as well as atrial and ventricular fibrillation

Potassium is an important key in maintaining the heart's normal electrical activity. When there is a greater than normal level of potassium in the blood, the myocardial excitability becomes reduced, resulting into weakened reaction of the conducting and pacemaking heart tissues.

When this condition worsens, the SA node's impulses become suppressed, and the AV node and His-Purkinje reduce conduction activities. This ultimately leads to conduction blocks, bradycardia, and even cardiac arrest.

The earliest sign of hyperkalaemia is peaked T waves. This implies repolarization aberrations.

When the atria become paralyzed, the P wave becomes wider and more flat, and the PR segments lengthen until they disappear altogether.

When the condition progresses, QRS intervals become prolonged and QRS complexes take on bizarre shapes. There may be high-grade AV blocks, accompanied by slow ventricular and junctional escape rhythms. Conduction blocks may also be present.

Slow AF or sinus bradycardia may be observed.

The ECG may develop a sine wave pattern, which is a danger sign. If this leads to cardiac arrest, ventricular fibrillation and asystole may occur.

Treatment

Limiting dietary intake and increasing excretion by using diuretics is sufficient for patients with moderate hyperkalemia without any ECG abnormalities. It is necessary to be vigilant with patients that have an AV block or bradyarrhythmia, especially those who have renal failure or on haemodialysis and taking potassium-sparing diuretics, ACE inhibitors, and potassium supplements. These things may cause a spike in potassium in the blood.

Hyperkalemia is treated by infusing calcium, in order to prevent cardiac arrest. Insulin-glucose infusion is given to drive potassium into cells. Loop diuretics are used to remove excess potassium. Metabolic acidosis, if present, is corrected by bicarbonate infusion.

Hyperthyroidism

The thyroid produces hormones that regulate how cells use energy. When it is hyperactive, it makes too much of these hormones, which creates unpleasant symptoms such as irregular heartbeat, fatigue, insomnia, and weight loss.

In the ECG, hyperthyroidism creates the following changes because of the increased responsiveness of the sympathetic nervous system and overstimulation of the myocardium:

> » Sinus tachycardia
>
> » Atrial fibrillation
>
> » Rapid ventricular response

» High voltage from left ventricles

» Supraventricular arrhythmias

» Ventricular extra systoles

» T wave and ST abnormalities

Treatment

Hyperthyroidism is treated by anti-thyroid medications, radioactive therapy, or thyroidectomy. Anti-thyroid medication includes propylthiouracil and methimazole, which inhibit the conversion of T4 to T3. Radioactive iodine (I131) is administered orally, and it is preferentially taken up by the thyroid gland, where it causes fibrosis and destruction of cells. Surgery can also be done for thyroid hormone-producing tumors.

Hypocalcemia

For the normal functioning of the cells, calcium must be present in appropriate levels in the blood. If there is a low amount of it, it will affect the way the cells work, including those in the heart.

The causes of hypocalcemia may be hypoparathyroidism (underactive parathyroid), vitamin D deficiency, hypomagnesemia, hyperphosphatemia, acute pancreatitis, diuretics, certain congenital diseases such as DiGeorge syndrome, and sepsis.

Symptoms are seizures, neuromuscular excitability, tetany, carpopedal spasm, Trousseau's sign, and Chvostek's sign.

ECG reflects prolonged QTc segments, specifically on the ST segments. The T wave is usually normal. Dysrhythmias are usually uncommon, but atrial fibrillation may sometimes occur. Torsades de pointes may also happen, but it is less likely as with hypomagnesaemia or hypokalaemia.

Treatment

Calcium and magnesium are given orally and intravenously. Mild hypocalcemia requires oral supplementation. Severe forms require IV infusion. Magnesium aids in calcium absorption. If seizures present, they are managed with benzodiazepines. If it is caused by other conditions such as hypoparathyroidism, these are treated.

Hypokalemia

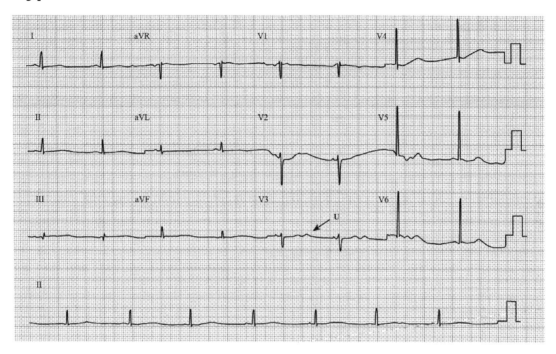

Figure 15. Hypokalemia is associated with small or absent T waves, prominent U waves, AV block, and slight ST depression.

Potassium regulates the electrical conduction of the heart. Decreased levels of potassium in the blood cause hyper-excitability of the heart cells, which leads to the development of re-entrant arrhythmias. This is often linked to hypomagnesaemia.

The effect of early hypokalaemia on the ECG causes the following features:

> » Bigger and longer P waves
> » Prolonged PR intervals

» Flat and inverted T waves

» Depressed ST segments

» Prominent U waves especially in the precordial leads

» Fusion of the T and U waves, causing what seems to be longer QT intervals

When it worsens, the ECG reflects these:

» Frequent supraventricular and ventricular ectopic beats

» Supraventricular tachyarrhythmias

» Ventricular arrhythmias

Treatment

Intravenous potassium is infused slowly at a rate of 10 mEq per hour. Continuous ECG monitoring is essential. The cause for hypokalemia must be diagnosed nd addressed; this may involve stopping diuretics and replacing with potassium sparing diuretics, and prevention of nausea, vomiting and polyuria.

Surgical intervention is required only in case of renal artery stenosis, intestinal obstruction, and adrenal adenoma.

Hypomagnesemia

Hypomagnesemia is the condition of having low levels of magnesium in the blood. This can happen because of malnutrition, alcoholism, diarrhoea, digestive disorders, excessive sweating, antibiotic and diuretic side effects.

The main sign of hypomagnesaemia in an ECG is a prolonged QTc segment.

Other than that, there is ectopy in the atria and ventricles, torsades de pointes, and tachyarrhythmia in the atria.

Treatment

Treating this involve correcting the serum magnesium levels. Intravenous magnesium is given at the rate of 50 mEq over 8 to 24 hours. Calcium and potassium levels must also be monitored and corrected if required. In case of torsades de pointes, 2mg magnesium rapid IV bolus is given.

Hypothermia

Hypothermia is body temperature that is below acceptable levels, usually below 35 degrees Celsius.

ECG clues of hyperthermia include shivering artefact (fuzzy ECG baseline), bradyarrhythmias (sinus bradycardia, slow junctional rhythms, atrial fibrillation with slow ventricular response, and AV blocks), ventricular ectopic beats, prolonged PR, QT, and QRS intervals, and Osborn waves (positive deflection at the J point in most leads except in aVr and V1, where they are negative). If unmanaged, it may trigger VT or VF. Sometimes, this can also lead to cardiac arrest.

Treatment

The hypothermic patient is warmed, using hot water bottles or chemical warmers, to regain normal body temperature. Lignocaine can be used to prevent cardiac dysrhythmias. If ventricular fibrillation occurs, chemical conversion could be attempted with intravenous bretylium, and supported by CPR when necessary. Defibrillation should be done when the patient's body temperature is above 30 degrees celsius to be effective.

Hypothyroidism

An underactive thyroid or myxoedema causes the body to produce minimal amounts of a hormone called thyroxin, which affects the ability of the heart to function properly.

In an ECG reading, hypothyroidism may be diagnosed with bradycardia, low QRS voltage, and widespread T-wave inversions, often without ST segment deviations.

Other supporting indicators are first degree AV block, QT segment prolongation, and intraventricular conduction delay.

These ECG abnormalities may be due to gelatinous connective tissue deposits in the myocardium, decreased sympathetic nervous system activity, and decreased chronotropy and inotropy of the heart.

Treatment

Synthetic thyroid hormone such as levothyroxine is given orally to treat hypothyroidism, at a starting dose of 50-75 µg per day. . Once the levels have been stabilized, patients should be carefully monitored for the signs of overdose such as palpitations, tachycardia, headache, fatigue, tremors, or angina.

I

Interventricular Conduction Delay (QRS widening)

This is when the duration of the QRS complexes exceed 100 ms, and there is a supraventricular rhythm.

This is most often caused by left ventricular hypertrophy or a bundle branch block.

Hyperkalaemia and TCA poisoning are the most significant causes of this condition.

Other causes include the following: Left anterior/posterior fascicular branch block, left/right bundle branch block, bifascicular block, trifascicular block, left ventricular/right ventricular hypertrophy, biventricular hypertrophy, dilated cardiomyopathy, Wolff–Parkinson-White syndrome, arrhythmogenic right ventricular dysplasia (AVRD), and Brugada syndrome.

Treatment

The cause of the interventricular conduction delay must be ascertained by thorough cardiac evaluation. Treatment is given according to the underlying cause. Treatments of the various causes are described in their respective sections.

Intracranial haemorrhage

Intracranial haemorrhage is bleeding within the skull, which can cause increased intracranial pressure. This is a dangerous condition that affects several parts of the body, including the heart's conduction system.

This is caused by traumatic brain injury, cerebral metastases, and massive ischemic stroke.

This is associated with bradycardia (Cushing reflex –warns of likely herniation of the brainstem), QT prolongation, widespread huge T-wave inversions (aka cerebral T waves).

Other ECG signs are:

» ST depression or elevation

» Increased amplitude of U waves

» Rhythm disturbances – atrial fibrillation, premature ventricular contractions, sinus tachycardia

Treatment

Intracranial haemorrhage requires intensive care in a medical facility. Endotracheal intubation is done to protect the airway, and hypotension is induced to a mean arterial pressure less than 130 mm Hg. Emergency CT scan should be performed after the vital signs have been stabilized. Intracranial pressure is monitored. Mannitol can be administered to control intracranial pressure. Normotonic fluids should be used to maintain brain perfusion without causing edema. Large hematomas must be evacuated surgically.

Intrinsicoid Deflection/ R Wave Peak Time

This is the time from the beginning of the earliest Q or R wave, up to the peak of the R wave in the lateral leads (V5 to V6, aVL),

This represents the time that it takes for the impulse to spread from endocardium to epicardium of the left ventricle.

The intrinsicoid deflection is said to be prolonged if it exceeds 45 ms.

Causes of this include left ventricular hypertrophy, left anterior fascicular block, and left bundle branch block.

Treatment

Intrinsicoid deflection is a symptom of an underlying condition.

This must be determined by thorough cardiac evaluation, and treated according to the cause as described in the individual sections.

J

J-point elevation

(See Benign Early Repolarization)

Junctional ectopic beat / junctional premature beat / Premature Junctional Contraction

It is a premature beat in the AV node. It appears rarely, but can have a regular grouped pattern, such as in cases of supraventricular bigeminy or trigeminy. This causes an irregular rhythm. The P wave is variable – it may be absent or be antegrade (appearing before the QRS complex) or retrograde (appearing after it). The PR interval is very short and the P-wave axis is abnormal or inverted in leads II, III, and aVF).

Treatment

No treatment is required if the patient is asymptomatic. If the patient presents with symptoms, the underlying cause is managed. The primary goal should be to decrease the rate by treating acidosis or electrolyte imbalances. Anti-arrhythmic medications such as amiodarone may be recommended. If it occurs because of digoxin, the drug is discontinued and counteracted. Caffeine may cause this as well. If so, caffeine intake is reduced.

Junctional Escape Beat

An escape beat results when the normal pacemaker does not fire, and the next pacemaker activates. The distance of the escape beat is always longer than the normal P-P interval.

This has an irregular rhythm. The P wave may be variable – it may be absent, antegrade, or retrograde. If it exists, it has a P-QRS ratio of 1:1. The PR interval may be non-existent, short, or retrograde. If it exists, it does not signify the atrial stimulation of the ventricles. QRS width is normal. There are no groupings but there are dropped beats.

Treatment

Treatment depends on the underlying cause/s of the junctional escape beat. If asymptomatic, this does not require treatment. If the beat is greater than 60 BPM, beta blocker such as esmolol may be used. Atropine or digoxin immune Fab may be used if junctional escape beat is caused due to digitalis toxicity. A permanent pacemaker may be indicated in patients presenting with complete AV block or sick sinus syndrome to speed up the ventricular rate and help normalize the arrhythmia.

Junctional Rhythm

A junctional rhythm is created as an escape rhythm, when the SA node and the atria's pacemaker do not function. It can occur during AV dissociation or third-degree AV block.

The rate is 40-60 BPM and regular. The P wave may be variable (absent, retrograde, or antegrade). The P:QRS ratio may be absent or 1:1. The PR interval may be non-existent, brief, or retrograde – if present, it does not represent the atrial stimulation of the ventricles. QRS width is normal and there are no grouping or dropped beats.

Treatment

The underlying cause of the junctional rhythm is corrected. Generally this condition may be physiological, and may not require treatment. However, if it is accompanied by dizziness and syncope, or it is associated with systemic comorbidities such as coronary artery disease, a pacemaker can be used to normalize the rhythm. If the junctional rhythm is due to digitalis toxicity atropine and digibind may be given. The junctional rhythm should not be suppressed though, because doing so may cause the ventricles to stop.

L

Lateral STEMI

Lateral STEMI is ST segment elevation myocardial infarction of the lateral portions of the heart.

This is recognizable by the ST elevation in the lateral leads (leads I, aVl, and V5 to V6) and corresponding ST depression in the inferior leads (leads III and aVF).

Treatment

Treatment for Lateral STEMI is the same as with myocardial infarctions. The first line of treatment for patients with STEMI is reperfusion by either mechanical (primary percutaneous intervention) or pharmacological interventions. Initial therapy is done with aspirin, morphine, and nitroglycerin. Intravenous access and supplemental oxygen should be provided immediately. Fibrinolytic therapy is started and surgery may be carried out for reperfusion.

Lead reversals: Limb Lead Reversals (overview)

This is simply the unintentional misplacement of limb lead electrodes. This may produce wrong readings that resemble heart diseases such as myocardial infarction/ischemia, chamber hypertrophy, and ectopic atrial rhythm.

Lead Reversal: Left Arm/Right Arm

LA/RA reversal may copy dextrocardia, but in contrast to the genuine illness, reversal has a normal R wave progression within the precordial leads.

Because the Einthoven's triangle are rotated 180 degrees, the Wilson's central terminal sends a zero signal, and the limb leads may look like other leads or become a flat line.

This results into the following disruptions:

» Lead I is inverted

» Leads II and III take each other's place

» Lead aVR and aVL switch

» Lead aVF is unchanged

» To determine RA/LL reversal, check the following:

» Lead aVR is upright

» Leads I to III and aVF are inverted (inverted P and T waves and QRS complexes)

Lead Reversal: Right Arm/Left Leg

Switching the RA and LL electrodes rotates the Einthoven's triangle 180 degrees vertically around the aVL axis.

This causes the following ECG effects:

» Inverted Lead II

» Inverted and reversed Lead I and III

» Switched aVF and aVR

» Unchanged aVL

To determine RA/LL reversal, look for these:

» Inversion of Leads I to III and aVF

» Upright aVR

RA/RL(N) reversal

Reversing the RA and RL(N) electrodes causes Einthoven's triangle to become a narrow triangle with the LA electrode at the apex.

The LL and LA leads record near identical voltages and makes their differences non-significant. The lead aVR faces opposite the lead II. Because the neutral electrode is displaced, aVF and aVL becomes identical and appears the same, but it will still be different to the baseline ECG.

So again, these are the indicators of RA/RL(N) reversal:

> » Lead III is a flat line (most obvious indicator)
>
> » Lead I = Lead II
>
> » Lead II is unchanged
>
> » Lead aVR is an inverted lead II
>
> » Lead aVL = Lead aVF

Bilateral Arm-Leg Reversal (RA-RL and LA-LL)

If the arm electrodes are switched with their associated leg electrodes (LL with LA and RL with RA), the Einthoven narrows down to a very small triangle with the LL electrode at the apex.

Because of this:

> » Lead I = flat line (most obvious indicator)
>
> » Lead II = inverted lead III
>
> » Lead III becomes inverted
>
> » aVR = aVL
>
> » aVF = negative lead III

LL/RL(N) Reversal

When the lower limb electrodes are reversed, Einthoven's triangle remains the same because the electrical signals from each leg are almost alike. This results to an unchanged ECG reading.

Treatment

Lead reversals do not require treatment. The position of the electrodes is verified, and if incorrect, electrodes are simply placed in their correct positions.

Left Atrial Enlargement / Left Atrial Hypertrophy

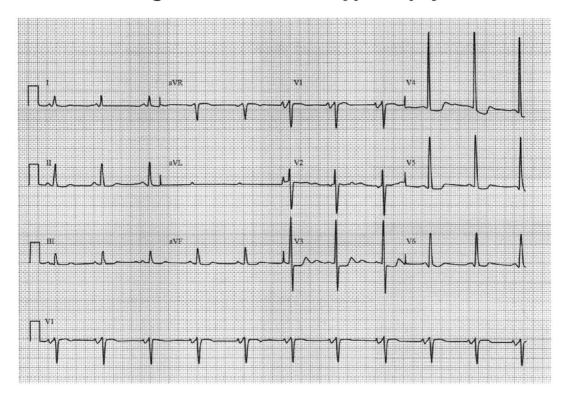

Figure 16. Left atrial abnormality (enlargement or hypertrophy) showing abnormal P waves (terminal negative components in lead V1)

The enlargement of the left atrium is caused by volume overload or pressure in it. This often causes atrial fibrillation.

This is often seen with mitral stenosis, and left ventricular hypertrophy (hypertrophic cardiomyopathy, aortic stenosis, mitral incompetence, and systemic hypertension).

This creates broad and bifid (M-shaped) P waves in lead II and bigger terminal negative portions of P waves in V1.

In particular:

» Lead II shows bifid P waves greater than 40 ms between two wave peaks, with total duration of greater than 110 ms.

115

» V1 shows biphasic P waves with terminal negative portions greater than 40 ms in duration and deeper than 1 mm.

Treatment

Left atrial enlargement is treated by addressing the underlying cause. Blood pressure should be managed through medications and dietary interventions. Beta blockers, ACE inhibitors, and diuretics can all help to control hypertension. Diuretics, anti-arrhythmics, and anti-coagulants should be given if the cause of enlargement is mitral stenosis. Surgical interventions such as mitral valve replacement should be considered only when other conservative options fail to respond. Electrical cardioversion and pacemaker implantation are performed if the underlying cause is atrial fibrillation.

Left Anterior Fascicular Block / Left Anterior Hemiblock

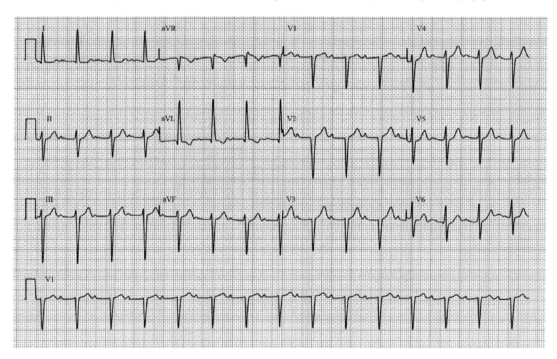

Figure 17. Left anterior hemiblock: LVH, LAH and long PR interval

Left anterior fascicular block is an electrical conduction abnormality, where impulses are carried through the left posterior fascicle and to the left ventricle.

LAFB ECG features are:

> » Left axis deviation (-45 to -90 degrees)
>
> » Small Q waves with tall R waves in Lead I and aVL
>
> » Small R waves with deep S waves in Lead II, III, and aVF
>
> » Increased QRS voltages in limb leads
>
> » Normal to slightly prolonged QRS (80-110 ms)
>
> » Prolonged R wave peak time in aVL that is greater than 45 ms

To distinguish LAFB from LVH, remember that in LAFB, the QRS voltage in the aVL lead will have no strain pattern in the left ventricle.

Treatment

There is no specific treatment for left anterior fascicular block, but it is a symptom of an underlying heart disorder. Therefore, a thorough cardiac evaluation is necessary to diagnose any underlying cardiac disease. If this disorder is causing unpleasant symptoms, treatment for the particular condition is given.

Left Axis Deviation

A left axis deviation is a description of QRS axis, that occurs between -30 and -90 degrees. It is caused by many conduction problems such as Wolff-Parkinson White syndrome, ventricular ectopy, left ventricular hypertrophy, left anterior fascicular block, left bundle branch block, inferior MI, and paced rhythm.

The following features are present when there is a left axis deviation:

> » QRS is positive and has dominant R waves in I and aVL.
>
> » QRS is negative and has dominant S waves in II and aVF.

Treatment

The cause for the left axis deviation is addressed. If the patient is asymptomatic, no treatment is required, apart from careful monitoring. Symptomatic patients require treatment according to the cause, as described in the respective sections.

Left Bundle Branch Block

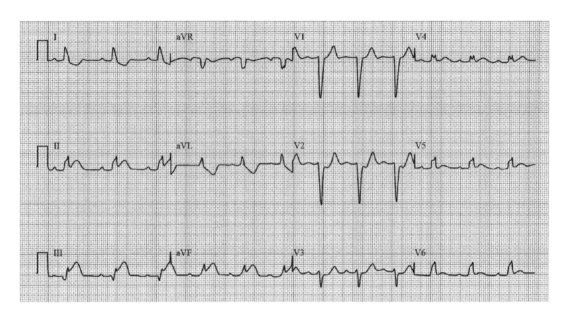

Figure 18. Acute myocardial infarction in the presence of left bundle branch block.

In LBBB, the septal depolarization becomes reversed (it goes from right to left instead of the usual left to right).

This is caused by various conditions like ischemic heart disease, aortic stenosis, anterior MI, dilated cardiomyopathy, fibrosis of the conducting system, hypertension, hyperkalaemia, and digoxin toxicity.

This aberration is indicated by the following features:

» QRS lasting longer than 120 ms

» Dominant S waves in V1

» Broad monophasic R waves in Leads I, avL, and V5 to V6

» No Q waves in I, V5 – V6

» R wave peak time is prolonged and measures greater than 60 ms in the left precordial leads V5 to V6

» ST segments and T waves go opposite the main vector of the QRS

» R waves progress poorly in precordial leads

» There is a general left axis deviation

In the lateral leads, the R wave takes on the following characteristics:

» Monophasic

» Notched

» M shaped

» Belongs to an RS complex

In V1, the following are observed:

» Small R waves, deep S waves

» Deep Q/S waves with no R wave before them

LBBB is described as incomplete when the QRS duration is less than 120 ms.

Reminder: LBBB is similar to LVH

Treatment

Treatment of this condition depends on the cause and the severity of the block. Patients who are asymptomatic generally do not require treatment, although they must undergo a cardiac evaluation, and be kept under observation. Patients who experience syncope-like symptoms would benefit from insertion of a pacemaker. If there is heart failure, cardiac resynchronization therapy must be done, which would regularize rhythm on both sides of the heart. A biventricular pacemaker should be considered for patients with prolonged QRS (>150ms).

Left Bundle Branch Block – How to Diagnose Myocardial Infarction (Sgarbossa Criteria)

The Sgarbossa criteria are standard ECG traits that are used to diagnose myocardial infarction when there is LBBB.

These are the updated criteria that should be witnessed in one or more leads:

» Concordant ST elevation measuring 1 mm or greater

» Concordant ST depression measuring 1 mm or greater in leads V1 to V3

» STE elevation measuring 1 mm or greater

» STE becoming more disorganized as based on 1/4th of the depth of the preceding S-wave

Treatment

Treatment for myocardial infarction is given as per guidelines. This includes initial therapy with aspirin, oxygen and nitroglycerin. Later management includes fibrinolytic therapy and surgical procedures to remove the block (CABG or angioplasty).

Left Main Coronary Artery Occlusion (ST Elevation In aVR)

The following ECG readings are indicative of this condition:

» ST elevation of 1mm or greater in aVR

» ST elevation in aVR is equal to or greater than in V1

» Widespread horizontal depression of the ST segments, most observed in I, II, and V4 to V6

Although the most prominent feature of left main coronary occlusion is ST elevation in aVR, this trait is also witnessed in other conditions: diffuse subendocardial ischemia after cardiac arrest, severe triple-vessel disease, and proximal left anterior descending artery occlusion

Treatment

This condition is considered as a STEMI equivalent, thus it is managed by emergent reperfusion therapy. CABG is considered the gold standard of therapy. However, percutaneous coronary interventions have also been carried out with equal success. This can be combined with imaging methods, such as intravascular ultrasound and optical coherence tomography, to improve results.

Left Posterior Fascicular Block / Left Posterior Hemiblock

In left posterior fascicular block, electrical impulses are carried to the left ventricle through the left anterior fascicle. This is less common than LAFB, because this is composed of a bundle of fibres. Remember that this condition may occur with an RBBB if there is a bifascicular block.

This creates the following ECG traits:

»   Right axis deviation that is greater than +90 degrees

»   Small R waves with deep S waves in leads I and aVL

»   Small Q waves with tall R waves in leads II, III, and aVF

»   Normal to slightly prolonged QRS duration measuring 80-110 ms

»   Prolonged R wave peak time in aVF

»   Increased QRS voltages in the limb leads

Remember to rule out other causes of right axis deviation before you diagnose LPFB.

Treatment

No treatment for this is given unless there are other underlying conditions, which are given appropriate treatments. The patient must undergo cardiac evaluation to find the extent of the condition. Physical exercise and dietary modifications can aid in improvement. However, if the condition progresses to a complete heart block, implantation of a pacemaker becomes essential.

Left Ventricular Aneurysm

An aneurysm in the left ventricle shows up as persistent elevation of the ST segments. This usually occurs after an acute myocardial infarction. However, it may also be caused by cardiac infections, cardiac myopathy, and congenital abnormalities.

This is believed to be caused by the paradoxical movement of the ventricular wall.

Key features of this are:

> » ST Elevation seen 2 weeks or more after an acute myocardial infarction
> » May have convex or concave morphology
> » Q- or QS waves are well formed
> » T waves are small compared to the QRS complexes
> » These traits are more easily seen in the precordial leads.

This is distinguished from acute STEMI as follows:

In left ventricular aneurysm, the new ECG is identical to the previous ones, the Q waves are well-formed, and there are no reciprocal ST depression and dynamic ST segment changes. The T-wave to QRS ratio is less than 0.36 in all precordial leads.

In acute STEMI, there are ECG changes compared to old ones, with the degree of ST elevation worsening, there is reciprocal ST depression, and there are STEMI symptoms such as chest pain, paleness, and hemodynamic instability. The T-wave to QRS ratio is greater than 0.36 in any precordial lead.

Treatment

Surgery is not necessary for majority of cases, but it is advised that the patient limit physical activity levels to avoid complications. Sometimes surgery may be performed for ventricular reduction. ACE inhibitors may also reduce the risk of aneurysm formation and left ventricular remodelling. Anti-coagulants are given to reduce the risk of thrombosis, while anti-arrhythmic agents are used to maintain rhythm.

Left Ventricular Hypertrophy

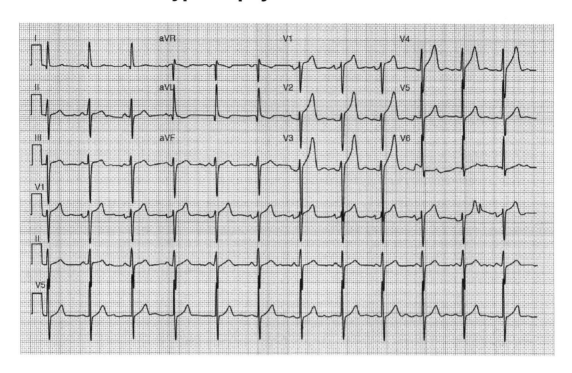

Figure 19. Left ventricular hypertrophy: increased QRS amplitudes and left axis deviation.

This is the enlargement of the left ventricle that may be caused by pressure overload in the chamber.

This is most frequently caused by hypertension but also by aortic regurgitation/stenosis, mitral regurgitation, hypertrophic cardiomyopathy, and aortic coarctation.

ECG changes pointing to LVH are numerous:

» Sokolov-Lyon criteria, which says that the S wave depth in V1 plus the tallest R wave height in leads V5 to V6 is greater than 35 mm

» R wave in lead I plus S wave in lead III is greater than 25 mm

» R wave in aVL is greater than 11 mm while in aVF is greater than 20 mm

» S wave in aVR is greater than 14 mm

» R wave in V4, V5, or V6 is greater than 26 mm

» R wave in V5 or V6 plus the S wave in V1 is greater than 35 mm

» The tallest R wave plus the tallest S wave in the precordial leads is greater than 45 mm

» Left axis deviation

» Left atrial hypertrophy indicators

» St elevation in the right precordial leads (V1 to V3) that are discordant to deep S waves

» Prominent U waves that are proportional to the increased QRS amplitudes

Treatment

Left ventricular hypertrophy is treated depending on the cause. If the patient is hypertensive, blood pressure reducers are used along with dietary intervention. These include ACE inhibitors, beta blockers, calcium channel blockers and diuretics. Sleep apnea, if present, must be treated witn cPAP. If aortic valve stenosis is the cause, surgery is undertaken to replace the aortic valve.

Lown Ganong Levine syndrome

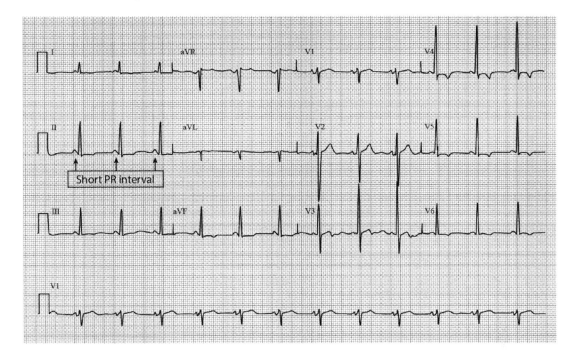

Figure 20. Lown Ganong Levine Syndrome depicting short PR interval and no delta waves.

This is a theoretical pre-excitation syndrome that involves an accessory pathway consisting of James Fibres. It is always associated with paroxysmal tachycardia.

ECG indicators are PR intervals of less than 120 ms and a normal QRS morphology.

Treatment

There is no particular treatment indicated for this syndrome. If there are symptoms, treatments to manage those symptoms are given. For instance, if the patient has tachycardia, pharmacological therapy for the same is instituted, such as beta blockers, calcium channel blockers, and digoxin. If medical therapy is ineffective, and patient has severe symptoms, pacemaker implantation or radiofrequency ablation may be considered.

Low QRS voltage

The voltage of the QRS segment is considered to be low when all amplitudes in the precordial leads are less than 10 mm, and are less than 5 mm in the limb leads.

These are generally caused by the loss of function in the myocardium, diffuse infiltration in the heart, or layers of fat, fluid, or air between the heart and the electrode.

The most significant cause is massive pericardial effusion, which causes tachycardia and electrical alternans aside from QRS with low voltages.

Treatment

Since low QRS voltage may be caused by different factors, the origin is determined and treated accordingly. Pericardial and pleural effusion are treated surgically by drainage. Cardiac tamponade needs to be treated with pericardiocentesis. COPD would require extensive medical therapy. If needed, thyroid and pulmonary function testing must be done in addition to cardiac workup.

M

Movement Artefact

This is caused by shivering or tremors. This is usually considered as a hindrance to accurate diagnosis, but it can be helpful for detecting hypothermia.

Certain conditions can cause this kind of artefact: anxiety, cerebellar disease, Parkinson's disease, benign essential tremor, thyrotoxicosis, drug toxicity, and drug withdrawal. Cardiopulmonary resuscitation may also cause this artefact.

Keep in mind that even simple talking and moving can cause the ECG to register a movement artefact. Thus the patient should be instructed to keep still and quiet during the procedure.

Treatment

This does not require treatment. The ECG may be repeated after some time to ensure an artefact-free reading from which a proper diagnosis can be made.

Multifocal atrial tachycardia

This is a tachycardia, Wandering Atrial Pacemaker. MAT and WAP are frequently linked with severe lung disease. This condition needs prompt treatment to prevent cardiovascular instability.

Heart rate is 100 BPM or higher. It has an irregularly irregular rhythm. The P wave may present as at least 3 different kinds. The P:QRS ratio is 1:1. The PR Interval is variable. QRS width is normal, and there are no grouping or dropped beats.

Treatment

The primary goal should be identification and treatment of the underlying cause. The ABCs should be stabilized and intravenous isotonic sodium chloride should be administered immediately. Bronchodilators and oxygen should be administered to treat COPD. Activated charcoal may be used if the cause is theophylline toxicity and it is indicated. Valsalva manoeuvre or carotid sinus massage may be done. Calcium channel blockers and beta blockers may be used to help normalize arrhythmia. Radiofrequency ablation and pacemaker implantation are considered in patients with recurrent MAT.

Myocardial Ischemia

Myocardial ischemia is a dangerous condition that is caused by the obstruction of the coronary artery.

It is considered as Non ST elevation myocardial infarction.

Major ECG signs include depression of the ST segments, and inversion (at least 1mm deep and present in two or more leads with dominant R waves) or flattening of T waves.

A unique ECG reading for myocardial ischemia is when the ST depression is horizontal, or slopes downwards for 0.5 mm or more at the J-point in two or more adjacent leads. Upsloping ST also indicates myocardial ischemia, but is not specific to it.

Additional signs are peaked T waves or pseudo-normalization of inverted T waves, and inversion of U waves.

The ECG signs will have some variations depending on the affected part:

» Subendocardial: widespread ST depression usually in leads I, II, V4 to V6

» Left main coronary artery occlusion: widespread ST depression

Treatment

Myocardial ischemia is treated by medications that open the arteries, help relax the heart muscle, and lower blood pressure such as aspirin, calcium channel blockers, beta blockers, nitrates, ACE inhibitors, and ranolazine. Anticoagulants may also be given to help remove blood clots. Surgery to improve the blood flow may be performed, such as angioplasty, stenting, and coronary artery bypass. Careful monitoring is essential to avoid infarction.

Myocarditis

Myocarditis is inflammation of the myocardium, without the presence of ischemia. This is usually benign but it can sometimes lead to dilated cardiomyopathy, arrhythmias, cardiogenic shock, and cardiac failure.

This is caused by bacterial and viral infections, immune reactions, toxins, and drugs.

ECG indicators for myocarditis are sinus tachycardia, ventricular arrhythmias, AV conduction aberrations, QRS or QT prolongation, and diffuse T wave inversion. This may also occur with pericarditis.

Treatment

Myocarditis is treated with medications that are commonly used for heart failure. These include diuretics, nitroglycerin, and ACE inhibitors. Anticoagulants may be given as a preventive measure. To reduce heart inflammation, steroids and similar drugs are given. Ventricular assist devices, intra-aortic balloon pump, and extracorporeal membrane oxygenation may be performed in severe cases. For serious myocarditis complications, a defibrillator or pacemaker may be used. It is important to withdraw the causative agent (eg. Drugs).

N

Non-Paroxysmal Junctional Tachycardia

(see accelerated junctional rhythm)

P

Pericardial Effusion/Tamponade

Pericardial effusion is a dangerous accumulation of fluid in the space surrounding the heart. This can increase the pressure to the heart, and affect heart function adversely.

This condition produces three effects: low voltage ECG readings, tachycardia, and electrical alternans.

Treatment

Tamponade is an emergency case that requires pericardiocentesis. In milder cases, pharmacotherapy may be used. Aspirin and steroids are useful for autoimmune conditions. Colchicine and antibiotics are also used. Afterwards, intravascular volume is expanded using blood, plasma, isotonic sodium chloride, or dextran. Inotropic drugs may assist in increasing cardiac output. The patient will also rest with legs elevated to help improve venous return.

Pericarditis

Pericarditis is the inflammation of the pericardium, or the membrane surrounding the heart.

This causes chest pain, fast heart beats, and difficulty breathing.

ECG indicators

» Widespread concave ST elevation and PR depression in most precordial and limb leads

» Reciprocal ST depression and PR elevation in the lead aVR

» Sinus tachycardia

» Pericardial effusion signs

It is possible to know the stage of pericarditis, based on the ECG readings:

» Stage 1 – widespread ST and PR depression with reciprocal changes in the lead aVR

» Stage 2 – ST changes normalizes but there is generalized flattening of T waves

» Stage 3 - T waves become inverted

» Stage 4 – ECG normalizes

Treatment

If pericarditis is accompanied with pericardial effusion, the patient's heart is surgically decompressed via pericardiocentesis. There are many types of pericarditis and it is treated depending on the type:

Idiopathic/inflammatory: anti-inflammatory drugs help control heart inflammation, while pericardectomy may be done for recurrent cases

Infectious: the infection is treated by antibiotics, anti-fungals, or chemotherapy

Metabolic: those with renal failure are given haemodialysis, and those who have hypothyroidism are given thyroid hormone therapy.

Cardiovascular: anticoagulants and thrombolytic medications may be given, but these should be discontinued if pericardial effusion develops

Persistent ST Elevation (LV Aneurysm Morphology)

(see Left Ventricular Aneurysm)

Polymorphic Ventricular Tachycardia (PVT)

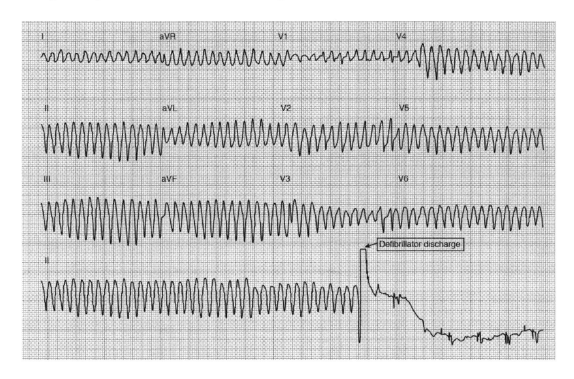

Figure 21. Polymorphic Ventricular Tachycardia (PVT), the rhythm strip shows the defibrillator discharge followed by pacemaker rhythm.

This is a particular kind of ventricular tachycardia with several ventricular foci. The most common cause of this is myocardial ischemia.

Torsades de Pointes is one form of PVT – for it to be considered as such, the PVT and QT segments should both be prolonged. Bidirectional VT is also a PVT type.

Treatment

Usually, this condition is self-limited. If it does not convert spontaneously, defibrillation must be done. The condition causing PVT is treated to prevent recurrence. Potassium and magnesium levels must be monitored and corrected. Surgical intervention such as ventricular reduction may be done. ACE inhibitors can also reduce the aneurysm. Lignocaine administration may be beneficial.

Poor R Wave Progression (PRWP)

This describes R waves that are 3mm or shorter in V3.

This feature is caused by conditions such as anteroseptal MI, left ventricular enlargement, and dilated cardiomyopathy. This may also be the result of misplacing V1 and V3. This may also be normal to a person.

Treatment

The condition causing the PRWP is identified and managed. These can include left bundle branch block, left anterior fascicular block, Wolff-Parkinson-White syndrome, and ventricular hypertrophy. The management of these conditions follow the same principles as described in the respective sections. If the person is asymptomatic, it may be normal and thus need not be treated.

Posterior STEMI

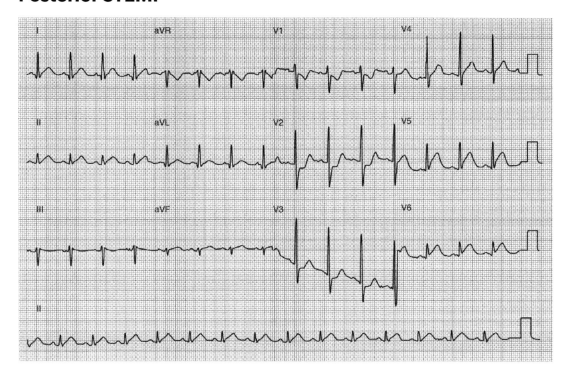

Figure 22. Acute posterior myocardial infarction is associated with tall R and upright T waves in lead V1-3.

This is the ST-Elevated Myocardial Infarction of the posterior (back) areas of the heart.

When a posterior STEMI is accompanied by lateral or inferior STEMI, the patient is in danger of a fatal left ventricular dysfunction. Thus, if a patient has an inferior or lateral STEMI, check for posterior STEMI as well.

To diagnose posterior STEMI, look for

- » Horizontal ST depression
- » T waves that are upright
- » Dominant R waves that measure greater than 30 ms and has an R to S ratio of greater than 1 in V2

Treatment

Posterior STEMI treatment is handled like any myocardial infarction case. Initial management is done with aspirin, oxygen, nitroglycerin, and morphine. Fibrinolytic therapy must be instituted as soon as possible. Coronary bypass grafting or percutaneous transluminal coronary angioplasty is done to re-establish circulation.

Preexcitation

This means early activation of the ventricles, because the impulses skip the AV node and head to the ventricles through an accessory pathway/bypass tract. This is commonly seen in Wolff-parkinson_white syndrome.

Treatment

Preexcitation syndrome has various manifestations. It is treated according to the severity and particular type of condition that has manifested. Acute tachyarrhythmias must be monitored, with oxygen supplementation and cardioversion. Management ideally includes radiofrequency ablation of the accessory pathway causing the pre-excitation. Anti-arrhythmic agents may be used to lessen the severity of symptoms.

Premature Ventricular Contraction (PVC)

PVC happens when a ventricular cell fires prematurely, or earlier than the SA node or supraventricular pacer. This causes the ventricles to be in a refractory state, that is, it's not yet repolarized and not ready to fire). The ventricles do not contract on the expected time. However, the beat after the PVC arrives on schedule, creating a compensatory pause.

PVC has an irregular rhythm. There is no P wave or P:QRS ratio on the PVC. There is no PR interval either. The QARS is wide (equal or greater to 0.12 seconds) and have a strange appearance. Groupings are usually absent, and there are 0 dropped beats.

Treatment

No treatment is needed if the patient does not have symptoms. If there are, PVC is treated according to the cause. Patients with mild symptoms can control them by lifestyle changes such as limiting caffeine and tobacco. PVC which has no other underlying condition is managed by medication such as lidocaine, amiodarone, and procainamide. Patients with severe symptoms, who do not respond to medical management, can undergo radiofrequency ablation.

Q

QRS widening

(See Intraventricular Conduction Delay)

Quetiapine Toxicity

Quetiapine is an anti-psychotic medication that can harm the heart in toxic doses. It can cause toxic coma, anticholinergic crisis and delirium, sinus tachycardia, and prolonged QTc.

Although the QTc is prolonged, this condition does not usually lead to Torsades de Pointes.

Treatment

Activated charcoal therapy at 1mg/kg, is started immediately to help remove the quetiapine. Wide bore IV access must be established, and intravenous sodium chloride solution is given to prevent hypotension. In case of seizures, benzodiapenes will help in controlling them. Ventricular dysrhythmias are treated with advanced cardiac life support and medications. If hyperthermia manifests, cooling measures must be undertaken. In order to reverse dopamine blockade, bromocriptine or amantadine may be given.

R

Right Atrial Enlargement/ Right Atrial Hypertrophy

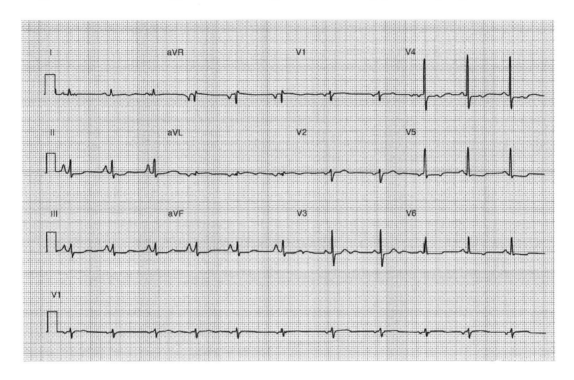

Figure 23. Right atrial hypertrophy showing tall and pointed
P waves (lead II).

This refers to enlargement of the right atrium. This is caused by chronic lung disease (eg. Cor pulmonale), primary pulmonary hypertension, congenital heart disease, and tricuspid stenosis.

Right atrial enlargement creates these ECG effects:

»   P waves greater than 2.5 mm in the inferior leads (II, III, aVF)

»   P waves greater than 1.5 mm in V1 and V2

Treatment

The condition causing the enlargement is treated. If the cause is pulmonary hypertension, whether primary or due to lung disease, anti-hypertensive medication is used. Surgery is indicated if the cause is a faulty tricuspid valve. Valve replacement is indicated in these cases.

Right Axis Deviation

This is a deviation of the QRS axis that measures somewhere between +90 and +180 degrees.

This is implied by the following ECG signs:

> » QRS is positive, and has a dominant R wave in leads aVF and III
> » QRS is negative, and has a dominant S wave in leads aVL and I

Following are the common causes of a right axis deviation: lateral myocardial infarction, ventricular ectopy, right ventricular hypertrophy, left posterior fascicular block, WPW syndrome, acute or chronic lung disease, sodium channel blocker toxicity, and hyperkalaemia.

This may also be normal for those with a horizontally-positioned heart.

Treatment

The cause of the right axis deviation must be identified and managed accordingly. If the deviation was not noted on previous ECGs, it could indicate exacerbated lung disease or pulmonary embolism. This requires a ventilation-perfusion scan, and anticoagulant therapy if needed. However, if the deviation is noted on serial ECGs, it could be a normal deviation, and may be observed periodically.

Right Bundle Branch Block

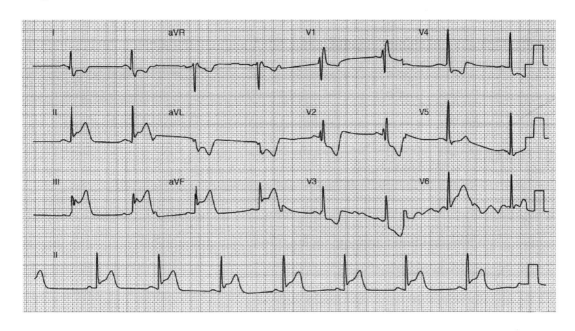

**Figure 24. Right Bundle Branch Block showing widened
QRS as well as secondary R waves (lead V1)**

RBBB happens when the right ventricle's activation is delayed because the depolarization is forced to travel across the septum to reach the left ventricle.

RBBB is a side-effect of ailments such as congenital heart disease, degenerative disease of the conduction system, ischemic/rheumatic heart disease, right ventricular hypertrophy, cor pulmonale, pulmonary embolus, cardiomyopathy, and myocarditis.

This abnormality causes the following ECG changes:

» Broad QRS segments measuring more than 120 ms

» RSR' pattern in V1 to V3 with M-shaped QRS complexes; if not, the R waves may be broad and monophasic in V1, forming qR complexes

» Wide (slurred) S waves in the lateral leads (I, aVL, and V5 to V6)

» T wave inversion and ST depression in the right precordial leads (V1 to V3)

Incomplete RBB

RBBB is described as incomplete when there is a pattern of RSR' in V1 to V3, with the QRS measuring less than 120 ms.

If the patient is a child, this pattern is often normal. It must be noted that this pattern may also be linked to Brugada syndrome, that is indicative of harmful ventricular arrhythmias.

Treatment

RBBB cases may be asymptomatic; if so, this does not require treatment. Follow up ECGs must be done every six months to assess for changes. However, if there is a pathological condition causing the RBBB, treatment is required to correct it. Medications that reduce high blood pressure and minimize the complications of heart failure are given. If needed, coronary angioplasty is done to open up a blocked artery causing the RBBB. A pacemaker can be implanted as well.

Right Ventricular Hypertrophy

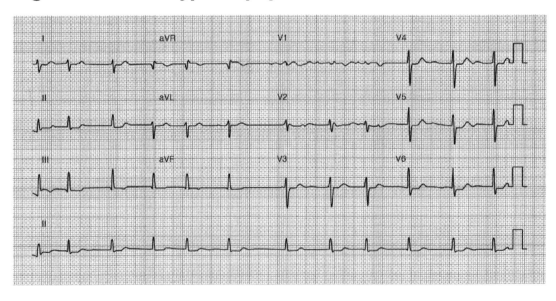

Figure 25. Right Ventricular Hypertrophy (irregularly irregular rhythm, absent P waves, and right axis deviation).

This condition signifies enlargement of the right ventricle, that may be caused by pulmonary embolism/hypertension, chronic lung disease, mitral stenosis, congenital heart disease, or arrhythmogenic right ventricular cardiomyopathy.

RVH may lead to RBBB.

This is diagnosed by the following conditions:

- » Right axis deviation that is +100 degrees or greater
- » Dominant R waves in V1 measuring greater than 7 mm in height, or with an R to S ratio of greater than 1
- » Dominant S waves in V5 or V6 measuring greater than 7 mm in depth, or with an R to S ratio of less than 1
- » QRS duration of less than 120 ms

Other signs that support this diagnosis are:

- » Right atrial hypertrophy
- » Right ventricular strain pattern, with ST depression, and T wave inversion in the inferior and right precordial leads
- » Deep S waves in the lateral leads
- » Far right axis deviation with dominant S waves in leads I to III

Treatment

The cause of the hypertrophy is managed. If pulmonary hypertension is present, vasodilator drugs such as epoprostenol are used. If the cause is systemic hypertension, ACE inhibitors, beta blockers and diuretics may be used. Surgical intervention is recommended in cases with structural defects, such as ventricular septal defects. Pacemakers are use in cases with rhythm alterations..

Right Ventricular MI

This is myocardial infarction that occurs in the right ventricle.

In right ventricular MI, RV contractility is poor, causing a heightened sensitivity to the preload. Because of this, preload-reducing agents can cause severe hypotension among patients with right ventricular MI.

This condition is treated with fluid loading.

To diagnose right ventricular MI in the patient, the following are checked:

» In general, the ST segments are elevated in the right leads (V3R to V6R)

» ST elevation in V1 + ST depression in V2 is equal (this is a very specific pattern for right ventricular MI)

» ST elevation in V1

» ST elevation in lead III is greater than in lead II, and it is greater in V1 than in V2

Treatment

During initial therapy, both nitroglycerin and morphine must be avoided as they are vasodilators. Fentanyl is given instead. Inotropics and thrombolytic therapy can help normalize right ventricular MI. Dopamine and dobutamine are used as vasopressors, and IV normal saline is given to maintain cardiac output. If there is a left ventricular dysfunction as well, an intra-aortic balloon pump and/or an infusion of nitroprusside help with reducing the afterload. A pacemaker may be installed when necessary.

Right Ventricular Outflow Tract (RVOT) Tachycardia

This is a kind of monomorphic ventricular tachycardia, that arises from the right ventricle's outflow tract, and sometimes from the tricuspid annulus.

The characteristics of RVOT tachycardia are: heart rate of greater than 100 BPM, LBBB morphology, QRS duration of greater than 120 ms, atrioventricular dissociation, and rightward or inferior axis measuring approximately +90 degrees.

Treatment

Patients without cardiac problems may have this pattern, but it is also witnessed among those with arrhythmogenic right ventricular dysplasia. The clinical course of this disease is benign and usually requires no treatment. For normal patients with mild symptoms,, this may respond to adenosine medication. Anti-arrhythmic agents are used in patients with severe symptoms; particularly those with arrhythmogenic RV dysplasia. Patients who do not respond to drugs may require more intensive treatments, such as radiofrequency ablation.

Right Ventricular Strain

This is an abnormal repolarization, because of enlargement or dilatation of the right ventricle.

This may be caused by any of these conditions: pulmonary hypertension/embolism, mitral stenosis, chronic lung disease, congenital heart disease, or arrhythmogenic right ventricular cardiomyopathy.

ECG traits that are seen include ST depression and T wave inversion in the right precordial leads and inferior leads, especially in lead III.

Treatment

The cause of the strain is managed according to the underlying condition, treatments of which are described in the individual sections.

R-wave peak time

(See Intrinsicoid Deflection)

S

Shivering artefact

(see movement artefact)

Short QT Syndrome

This is an arrhythmogenic condition that presents with paroxysmal atrial and ventricular fibrillation and syncope, which may trigger sudden cardiac death.

Treatment

Patients who have survived cardiac arrest, or who have ventricular tachyarrhythmias with syncope, benefit from implantable cardioverter-defibrillator placement. Some anti-arrhythmic agents such as quinidine and hydroquinidine are also effective in dealing with this syndrome, as they prolong the QT interval. Patients who present with atrial fibrillation may be treated with propafenone.

Sinus Arrhythmia

This rhythm is not that significant, and often creates no symptoms. However, it can be detected as speeding up of the pulse while inhaling and slowing down upon exhaling. This kind of rhythm may stop when the heart rate increases during exercise.

Sinus arrhythmia is caused by several things such as drugs (morphine, digoxin), increased ICP (Intra-cranial Pressure), inferior MI, and reflex vagal activity inhibition. If it is observed during inhalation, it may be due to increased heart rate and/or venous return, or decreased vagal tone. During exhalations, it is possibly due to decreased heart rate and/or venous return, or increased vagal tone.

Treatment

Since this is a normal characteristic of the heartbeat, it is normally not treated. If the condition presents with other symptoms such as dizziness or loss of consciousness, the treatment is directed towards the cause of the symptoms.

Sinus Bradycardia

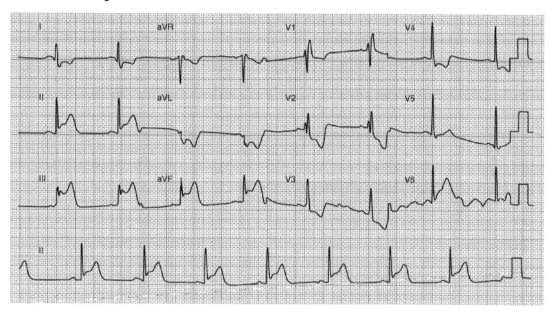

Figure 26. Sinus bradycardia, the rate is about 45 bpm

Sinus Bradycardia is characterised by a rate slower than 60 BPM. This may be caused by SA node or atrial pacemaker abnormalities, vagal stimulation, or medicines. Some athletes also have a slower heartbeat because their heart pumps blood efficiently.

The QRS complexes, PR, and QTc intervals may be normal or a bit prolonged. They should not exceed the upper limit for the normal range, however.

A person may have sinus bradycardia and experience no symptoms. In the case of symptoms, the cause of the bradycardia is treated with drugs such as epinephrine, dopamine, or atropine. A pacemaker may be inserted for severe cases.

Treatment

If asymptomatic, sinus bradycardia does not require treatment. If symptomatic, the underlying cause is treated, such as discontinuing drugs (e.g. Digitalis), and correcting hypothermia. Atropine may be given to improve perfusion. Long term prevention must be done by transcutaneous or transvenous pacing. While the pacer is not yet ready, or if it is ineffective, atropine or epinephrine/dopamine infusion is administered.

Sinus Pause / Arrest

The sinus pause is a time period when the sinus pacemaker is not working.

This may occur as a result of cardioactive drugs (digoxin, amiodarone, beta-adrenergic blockers, calcium-channel blockers, quinidine, and procainamide), acute infection, acute myocarditis, acute inferior-wall MI, cardiomyopathy, CAD, hypertension, sinus node disease, and increased vagal tone.

It is important to monitor the pulse and heart sounds during this condition, also to prepare against symptoms of decreased cardiac output such as low blood pressure, dizziness, altered mental status, and fainting.

If the pause is caused by medication, it should be discontinued. Symptoms are treated accordingly.

The rhythm is usually regular, except during the pauses. It is usually at 60-100 BPM before a pause occurs. When there are manypauses which are prolonged, the heart rate may slow down.

The pauses do not reflect the overall P-P intervals. There are dropped beats, but there is no grouping. The P wave may be absent in areas of pause or arrest, and QRS complexes may be missing as well. If present, it often comes before a QRS complex.

Treatment

The cause of the sinus pause is managed. If the cause is due to increased vagal tone, no treatment is required but the patient must be monitored. If it is caused by drugs, these are discontinued.

Potassium levels must be monitored and corrected if needed. A pacemaker may be inserted.

Sinus Tachycardia

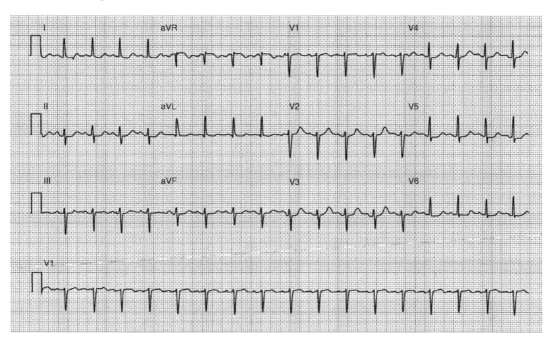

Figure 27. Sinus tachycardia, the rate is greater than 100 bpm

This is caused by conditions or medications that increase the output of the heart. For example, exercise, haemorrhage, hypovolemia (low blood volume), hypoxemia (low oxygen level in the blood), and acidosis.

The rhythm is regular. The P wave exists, and has a one to one ratio with the QRS. PR interval and QRS width may be normal to slightly shortened. There are no grouping or dropped beats.

The patient should be placed in a relaxed environment and be taught relaxation techniques to prevent worsening of the condition. This rhythm is also common after MI, and therefore an MI patient should have his/her heart rhythm monitored.

Treatment

If asymptomatic, sinus tachycardia is not treated. Lifestyle modifications such as avoiding caffeine and nicotine may be employed. Other triggers of the tachycardia are identified and eliminated. If caused by cardiac ischemia, beta-adrenergic blockers or calcium channel blockers are given.

Sodium Channel Blocker Overdose/Tricyclic Overdose

Sodium channel blockers, such as tricyclic antidepressants, type Ia and type Ic antiarrhythmics, local anaesthetics, propranolol, quinine, and carbamazepine, are harmful if taken in large doses.

Their main effects are ventricular dysrhythmias and seizures.

Blocking the sodium channels in the myocardium and the central nervous system results to the malfunction of the firing of cells, which will lead to symptoms such as the following:

- » Low blood pressure
- » Broad complex dysrhythmias
- » Tachycardia
- » Anticholinergic syndrome
- » Sedation
- » Coma

The ECG effects are the following:

- » QRS prolongation (greater than 100 ms can lead to seizures while greater than 160 ms can trigger ventricular arrhythmias)
- » Tall R waves in aVR

» Qtc prolongation because of the inhibition of the potassium channels

» Myocardial depression

Treatment

Caregivers need to ensure that the patient has a clear airway and can breathe adequately. Oxygen should be delivered at a high flow rate so that the patient is hyperventilated to maintain a ph level of 7.5-7.55. They should be ready to resuscitate the patient when needed.

Activated charcoal may be given to absorb and flush out the toxic substance from the body.

Seizures are treated with IV benzodiazepines, while hypotension is managed with a crystal bolus or vasopressors.

In case of arrhythmias, sodium bicarbonate is given. When pH is greater than 7.55, lidocaine is given intravenously.

Amiodarone, beta-blockers, procainamide and flecainide are prohibited, because they can worsen conduction problems and hypotension.

ST Elevation In AVR (Lmca/3vd)

(See Left Main Coronary Artery Occlusion)

STEMI

STEMI, Anterior

(See Anterior STEMI)

STEMI, high lateral

High lateral STEMI is detected in the high lateral leads I and aVL. There is reciprocal ST depression in the inferior leads III and aVF and V1 to V3.

T waves may be hyperacute in V5 to V6.

QS waves may have poor R wave progression in the anteroseptal leads V1 to V4.

STEMI, Inferior

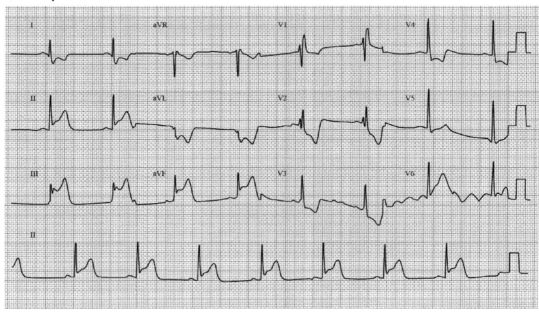

Figure 28. Acute inferior myocardial infarction characterized by ST elevation in inferior leads and reciprocal ST depression in anterior leads.

Inferior ST elevated Myocardial Infarction occurs in around half of STEMI cases. Some of them will also have a right ventricular infarction; they should not be given nitrates, to avoid hypotension. There are a few cases who will also have second or third degree AV block, causing them to have bradycardia – these are high risk cases. If inferior STEMI is accompanied with posterior infarction, there is a large area of myocardium involved, and this may be harder to treat.

This condition is caused by the blockage of the coronary arteries – the right coronary artery, the left circumflex artery, and/or left anterior descending artery.

The clues for inferior STEMI are ST elevation and Q wave development in the inferior leads (II, III, and aVF), and reciprocal ST depression in lead aVL.

To know which arteries are involved, these are considered:

The right coronary artery goes to the middle part of the heart's bottom wall, including the inferior septum – this creates an ST elevation in lead III that is greater than in lead II. There will also be a reciprocal ST depression in lead I. Indicators for right ventricular infarction are also likely to be present (ST elevation in leads V1 and V4R).

The left circumflex artery goes to the side of the heart's bottom wall and left posterobasal portion – producing ST elevation in leads I, aVL, and/or V5 to V6. The ST elevations in lead II is equal in lead III. There is no reciprocal ST depression in lead I.

As mentioned, inferior STEMI may manifest with bradycardia and AV blocks. This may be caused by AV node ischemia, because of impaired blood flow within the AV nodal artery and/or the Bezold-Jarisch reflex, which is an ischemia-related increase of vagal tone.

The blocks in inferior STEMI may begin as 1st degree AV block, linked to Wenckebach and progress to second/third degree AV block or complete heart block.

Sinus node abnormalities may show up as sinus pauses or arrests, sinus bradycardia, or sinoatrial exit block.

It is fortunate though that AV blocks and bradyarrhythmias in inferior STEMI are usually temporary, and can be managed with atropine.

STEMI, Lateral

Lateral ST elevated myocardial infarction involves the lateral (side) walls of the heart. This results from the blockage of the left anterior descending artery and left circumflex artery.

Lateral STEMI is a significant diagnosis, and this alone is enough to indicate emergent reperfusion.

If this exists with anterior, posterior, or inferior MI, it signifies that a large area of the heart is in danger, and it may be more difficult to treat.

Indications of lateral STEMI are ST elevation in lateral leads I, aVL, and V5 to V6, as well as reciprocal ST depression in inferior leads III and aVF.

STEMI (old)

(see Left Ventricular Aneurysm)

STEMI, Posterior

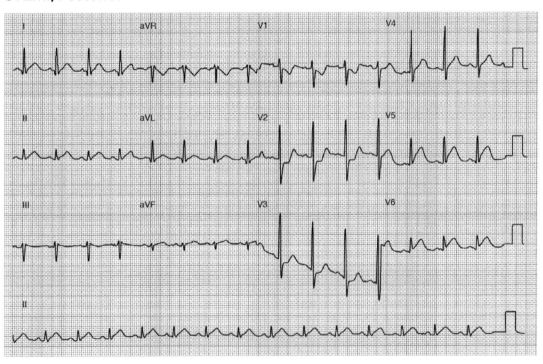

Figure 29. Acute posterior myocardial infarction associated with tall R waves and upright T waves in leads V1-3.

This occurs in less than 1/5 of STEMI cases, usually along with inferior or lateral infarction.

If there is an inferior and/or lateral infarction as well, posterior STEMI signifies injury of a large area of the heart. This increases the risk of left ventricular dysfunction and other fatal conditions. So, if there is a patient with lateral or inferior STEMI, always check for posterior MI as well.

Isolated posterior infarction indicates the need for emergent coronary reperfusion, but it is hard to diagnose, because ST elevation in this area is hard to detect. To know whether there is posterior infarction, check the leads V1 to V3 for the following traits:

- » Horizontal ST depression
- » Tall and wide R waves measuring greater than 30 ms and has R to S ratios of greater than 1 in V2
- » Upright T waves

STEMI, right ventricular

(see right ventricular MI)

Treatment

Treating all kinds of STEMI is similar to how myocardial infarction is treated. Emergency management includes administration of aspirin, nitroglycerin, and morphine, with supplemental oxygen. Fibrinolytic therapy must be started, and the patient must be taken up for surgery to establish reperfusion if required (CABG).

Subarachnoid Haemorrhage

(see raised intracranial pressure)

T

Tako Tsubo Cardiomyopathy

This is an ST elevated Myocardial Infarction, that resembles ischemic chest pain, but it is not caused by blocked coronary arteries. This is common among those who are experiencing emotional distress. It is called Tako Tsubo because the left ventricle appears like a Japanese basket (tsubo) that is used to catch octopi (tako).

This is common among emotionally distressed post-menopausal women. This phenomenon is theorized to be caused by a surge of catecholamine, which activates the nervous system and causes the blood vessels to spasm. Also, the presence of LVOTO (left ventricular outflow tract obstruction) may increase its likelihood.

Indicators:

> » There are new changes in the ECG readings, such as T wave inversion or ST elevation
>
> » Troponin may rise
>
> » The left ventricle may move abnormally, specifically in the centre and apex
>
> » There are no blockages in the coronary arteries

Although Tako Tsubo has similar ECG readings to STEMI, it is milder than the latter, but it still needs treatment.

Treatment

There are no specific guidelines for tako tsubo cardiomyopathy. Since this condition resembles STEMI on the first ECG, initial management would be the same. Once differentiated, however, heart failure medication like ACE inhibitors, beta blockers, and diuretics may help. Aspirin may also be given. Stress management plays an important role in management of this condition.

Torsades de Pointes

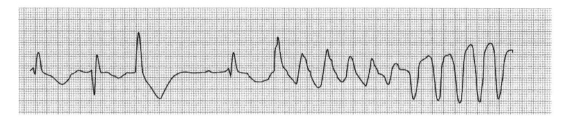

Figure 30. Polymorphous ventricular tachycardia (Torsade de Pointes) showing wide QRS complexes and changing R-R intervals.

Torsade de Pointes translates to twisting of points. It has an irregular rhythm that is at 200-250 BPM. Its main feature is its wavy appearance wherein the QRS complexes axis changes from positive to negative and back again randomly. It can revert to a normal rhythm, or fall into ventricular fibrillation, which can be fatal. There are no P waves, P:QRS ratios, PR Intervals, and dropped beats. The QRS width is variable, and the grouping has a variable sinusoidal pattern.

This is caused by several things: electrolyte imbalances, drug toxicity, myocardial ischemia, SA node diseases, and AV blocks.

Treatment

Immediate management includes administration of magnesium, which must be monitored carefully. Mexiletine may also be useful. Long term management of torsades de Pointes is managed by addressing the underlying cause. It may require cardiopulmonary resuscitation, defibrillation, and overdrive pacing. If the patient is unstable, synchronized cardioversion may be necessary.

Tremor Artefact

(see movement artefacts)

Tricyclic Overdose (Sodium-Channel Blocker Toxicity)

(see sodium-channel blocker toxicity)

Trifascicular Block

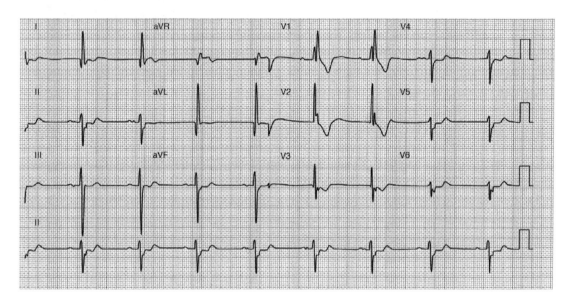

Figure 31. Trifascicular block (often a combination of RBBB, LAFB, and long PR interval).

This is the blockage of all three conducting fascicles of the heart:

> » Left anterior fascicle
>
> » Left posterior fascicle
>
> » Right bundle branch

Main causes are ischemic heart disease, aortic stenosis, anterior MI, conducting system disease, congenital heart disease, digoxin toxicity, and hyperkalaemia

This is classified into two:

Incomplete

This may lead to complete heart block but it's not that likely as a complete trifascicular block.

The most common of incomplete trifascicular block is a bifascicular block and a 1st degree AV block.

A bifascicular block may occur with a 2nd degree AV block as well.

A right bundle branch block may have an alternating Left Anterior Fascicle Block and Left Posterior Fascicular Block

Complete

This is a bifascicular block combined with a third degree AV block.

Treatment

The most recommended treatment for a trifascicular block is the insertion of a pacemaker.

V

Ventricular Aneurysm

(see left ventricular aneurysm)

Ventricular Escape Beat

This is similar to the junctional escape beat, but it occurs in the ventricles. This beat occurs when the ventricles do not receive adequate signal from the atria; so they initiate a beat on their own to prevent arrest. The pause is non-compensatory because the normal pacer did not fire. The pacer then resets itself and creates a new timing, which may have a different rate than before.

The rhythm of a ventricular escape beat is irregular. There are no P waves, thus no P:QRS ratios and PR intervals as well. The QRS width is wide (0.12 seconds or higher), and has a strange form. There are no groupings or no dropped beats.

Treatment

Since ventricular escape beat acts to prevent a cardiac arrest, treatment is not required. The cause of the escape beat must be identified, and that must be treated. For instance, if the ventricular escape beat is caused by a third degree AV block, it is treated with cilostazol, which will increase ventricular escape. Other than that, an ouabain infusion reduces ventricular escape time and increases ventricular escape rhythm.

Ventricular Escape Rhythm / Idioventricular Rhythm

This occurs when the primary pacemaker is a ventricular focus. Because it originates from the ventricles, the QRS complexes are wide and strange looking. This rhythm is regular and has a slow rate of 20-40 BPM. It can occur by itself or as a result of AV dissociation or third degree heart block. There are no P waves, P:QRS ratios, PR intervals, groupings, and dropped beats.

Treatment

Treatment is usually aimed at addressing the cause of escape rhythm. This is the last pacemaker, thus this is not treated with antiarrhythmics because doing so may stop the heart altogether. Instead, atropine can be used to increase the heart rate. A temporary or permanent pacemaker may be inserted to correct the rhythm for prolonged periods of time.

Ventricular Fibrillation (Vfib)

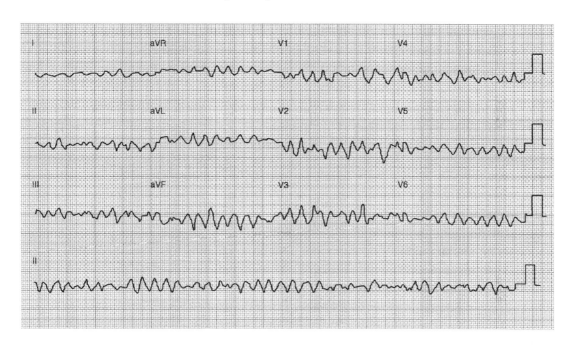

Figure 32. Ventricular fibrillation: a bizarre, irregular waveform with no clearly discernable P waves or QRS complexes.

When many areas of the heart are firing in a disorganized manner, it results in Ventricular Fibrillation. This has an indeterminate rate, and a chaotic rhythm. There are no beats at all, thus no P waves, QRS complexes, and so on.

VFib causes recognizable symptoms such as loss of consciousness, and absence of pulse. If the patient looks and acts normal, the leads may just have fallen off.

Treatment

Since this is a life threatening emergency, ACLS protocol is followed. Cardiopulmonary resuscitation, with defibrillation of 200 J are given for ventricular fibrillation. Simultaneously, 1 mg of epinephrine is given every 3 to 5 minutes. One dose of amiodarone, or upto three doses of lidocaine are also given.

In order to prevent VF in susceptible patients, implantable cardioverter defibrillators may be used. Radiofrequency ablation may be used in selected cases. Anticoagulant therapy is also given.

Ventricular Flutter

This is an extreme form of ventricular tachycardia, and quickly progresses to ventricular fibrillation. The beats come in at 200-300 BPM and there are no discernable P waves, QRS complexes, T waves, and T segments. It forms a regular sinusoidal pattern. There are no groupings and dropped beats.

A VFlutter at the rate of 300 BPM can indicate Wolff-Parkinson-White Syndrome with an atrial flutter of 1:1 conduction.

Treatment

Ventricular flutter is an emergency. As per ACLS protocols, CPR must be initiated immediately, and defibrillation must be done, using an external electric shock of 200-400 joules. This treatment is to be continued even if the patient progresses to ventricular fibrillation. Once the patient is stable, further recurrences are avoided by drugs such as amiodarone, procainamide, and lidocaine.

Ventricular Tachycardia (VTach)

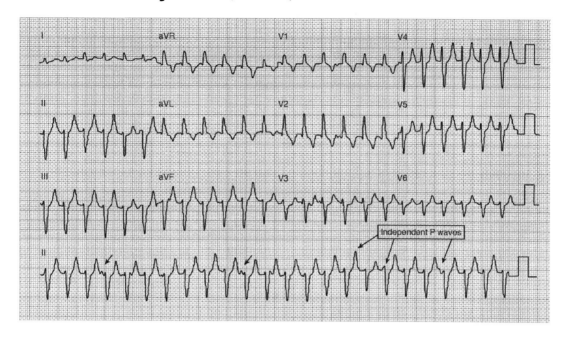

Figure 33. Ventricular tachycardia characterized by wide QRS complexes and AV dissociation (independent P waves).

This is a very rapid ventricular rate that is often separate from an underlying atrial rate. There are QRS irregularities at regular intervals, which represent underlying sinus beats. The P wave shows a dissociated atrial rate. P: QRS ratio is variable, and there is no PR interval. WRS width is wide and abnormal. Rhythm is regular and clocks at a speed of 100-200 BPM. There are no grouping or dropped beats. It is important to remember that wide QRS tachycardia is VT until proven otherwise.

Variations:

Fusion Beats

Sinus beats may sometimes allow the ventricle to become innervated through the normal ventricular conduction system.

This leads to a fusion beat – a blend of an abnormal ventricular beat and a normal QRS complex. This is created by two pacemakers working together, the SA node and the ventricular pacer.

Capture beats

A capture beat is completely innervated by the sinus beat, and cannot be distinguished from a normal complex. It occurs during VTach, and by luck, it beats at the right time to transmit through the AV node and depolarize the ventricles.

Ventricular Tachycardia can be diagnosed when there are fusion and capture beats. These are noticeable as a tachycardic rhythm with wide complexes. (total QRS is greater or equal to 0.16 seconds), and negativity of precordial leads (V1 to V6). Other indicators are as follows:

Brugada's Sign

This has an interval from the R wave to the bottom of the S wave, measuring 0.10 seconds or greater.

Josephson's sign

This is a small notching near the bottom point of the S wave.

It is a common error to mistake VTach for a supraventricular tachycardia. Consider it as VTach just to be safe.

Treatment

Ventricular tachycardia can manifest if there is no pulse; if so, ACLS guidelines must be instituted immediately. This includes CPR and defibrillation. If there is a pulse but the patient is unstable, synchronized cardioversion is performed immediately. Electrolyte imbalances are corrected if present. An ICD may be implanted for recurrent VT. Clinically stable patients are usually treated with anti-arrhythmic drugs.

Ventricular Tachycardia: Fascicular VT

Idiopathic VT is a ventricular tachycardia condition that occurs without structural abnormalities of the heart. Only around 10% of VT cases are idiopathic (without pathological cause), and up to 90% of these starts from the right ventricle.

Among idiopathic VT cases coming from the left ventricle, fascicular VT is the most common.

This condition happens among those who are young and healthy. It can be provoked by things that cause the heart to beat faster, such as stress, emotional distress, exercise, and some medications, but it can also happen while resting.

The possible cause of this is re-entrant tachycardia is an ectopic focus inside the left ventricle.

ECG features:

> » Monomorphic ventricular tachycardia indicators such as capture beats, fusion complexes, and AV dissociation
> » QRS duration of 100 – 140 ms (shorter than most VT forms)
> » Brief RS interval of 60 – 80 ms
> » RBBB pattern
> » Axis deviation

Fascicular VT is classified according to the location of the re-entry circuit

Posterior fascicular VT is the most common kind, occurring in up to 95% of cases. It has a RBBB morphology and left axis deviation. It originates near the left posterior fascicle.

Anterior fascicular VT: This accounts for up to 10% of cases. There is RBBB morphology and a right axis deviation. This begins near the left anterior fascicle.

Upper septal fascicular VT: This occurs in a minimal percentage of cases. It can show either an RBBB or LBBB morphology with narrow QRS complexes. The axis may also be normal. This occurs from the upper septum.

This can be misdiagnosed as SVT with a RBBB – to make a proper diagnosis, additional features are considered, such as AV dissociation and fusion or capture beats, which are particular in VT.

Treatment

Treatment of this condition depends on the severity of symptoms. For patients with severe symptoms, radiofrequency catheter ablation is the treatment of choice. In patients with mild to moderate symptoms, drug therapy is initiated. Managing this typically involves verapamil. If it is induced by digoxin, it is counteracted by Digoxin Immune Fab.

Ventricular tachycardia: Monomorphic VT

Monomorphic VT is caused by hypertrophic or dilated cardiomyopathy, ischemic disease, and Chaga's disease.

Indicators:

>   QRS complexes are very wide, measuring around 200 ms.

>   The axis may be indeterminate.

>   Fusion and capture beats may be present.

>   Josephson's sign may be seen, with notching near the S wave's nadir (best observed in leads II, III, and aVF)

>   Brugada's sign may also be seen with monomorphic VT – time from the beginning of QRS until the S wave's nadir is longer than 100 ms (this is more obvious in V6).

Treatment

Treatment is based on whether the patient is hemodynamically stable or unstable. Unstable patients would present with dyspnoea, hypotension, and altered level of consciousness. Such patients are immediately treated with synchronized direct current cardioversion, with a starting dose of 100 J. If the patient is stable and asymptomatic, with normal left ventricular function, the patient is given pharmacotherapy, which includes intravenous procainamide, sotalol, or lidocaine.

If left ventricular function is impaired, amiodarone or lidocaine is preferred over other medications. If it is caused by drug toxicity or electrolyte imbalances, these are addressed.

W

Wellens Syndrome

This is an ECG pattern that accurately diagnoses critical stenosis of the left anterior descending artery. Those with this sign are at risk of experiencing extensive anterior wall MI, even though there may be no symptoms present.

The criteria for Wellen's Syndrome are:

» Inverted or biphasic T waves in leads V2 to V3 or sometimes from V1 to V6

» Minimally elevated ST segments measuring less than 1 mm

» Q waves are absent in the precordial leads

» R waves progress in the precordial leads

Treatment

Wellen's syndrome must be monitored via serial ECGs because it does not usually present symptoms, and it may lead to myocardial infarction. If ST segment elevation is seen, treatment must be instituted immediately. This includes supplemental oxygen, aspirin, and nitroglycerin. Laboratory studies must be done to confirm or rule out MI. An angiography may also be done to evaluate whether the patient may need coronary bypass surgery or angioplasty.

Wolff-Parkinson-White Syndrome

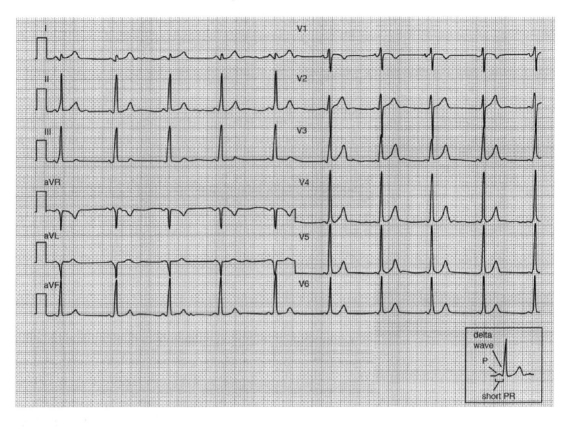

Figure 34. Wolf-Parkinson-White syndrome showing short PR interval, broad QRS with a slurred upstroke (delta wave), and secondary ST changes.

This syndrome is named after the people who discovered it: Louis Wolff, John Parkinson, and Paul Dudley White. It is a congenital condition where the heart has an accessory pathway that predisposes it to tachyarrhythmia.

The accessory pathway in WPW is the atrioventricular bypass tract (Bundle of Kent).

WPW indicators:

» PR interval is less than 120 ms

» There is a delta wave or slow rise at the beginning of the QRS segments

» The QRS measures greater than 110 ms

» The ST segment and T wave moves towards the opposite direction of the QRS segments' main components

» There is paroxysmal tachycardia

Localizing the accessory pathway

LOCATION	V1	V2	QRS AXIS
Left posteroseptal (type A)	+ve	+ve	Left
Right lateral (type B)	-ve	-ve	Left
Left Lateral (type C)	+ve	+ve	Inferior (90 degrees)
Right posteroseptal	-ve	-ve	Left
Anteroseptal	-ve	-ve	normal

Treatment

There are several treatment modalities depending on the underlying cause. The first-line treatment for symptomatic WPW is electrophysiologic study with radio-frequency catheter ablation. This can be done in conjunction with cryoablation. If the patient is at a high risk of ablation related complications, drug therapy may be used to treat WPW. Agents acting on the AV node, such as calcium channel blockers, beta blockers and digitalis may be used. Agents that act on the accessory pathway, such as quinidine and amiodarone, may also be used.

Exercises

1. A sign of Ventricular Tachycardia that means an interval from the R wave to the bottom of the S wave, measuring 0.10 seconds or grater.

    a. Josephson's sign

    b. Brugada's sign

    c. Capture beats

    d. Fusion beats

2. A condition that has a wavy appearance on the ECG, and has an irregular rhythm measuring 200-250 BPM.

    a. Normal Sinus Rhythm

    b. Bundle Branch Block

    c. Torsades de Pointes

    d. De Winter's T Waves

3. This toxicity causes bradycardia and AV block.

    a. Beta-blocker/calcium channel toxicity

    b. Digoxin toxicity

    c. Carbamazepine cardiotoxicity

    d. Quetiapine toxicity

4. A deviation of the QRS axis, measuring somewhere between +90 and +180 degrees.

    a. Right axis deviation

    b. Left axis deviation

    c. Extreme left axis deviation

    d. Extreme right axis deviation

5. A condition where the duration of the QRS complexes is greater than 100 ms and there is a supraventricular rhythm.

    a. Interventricular Conduction Delay

    b. Hyperkalemia

    c. Electrical Alternans

    d. Dextrocardia

6. The best way to treat a ventricular escape rhythm is to use anti-arrhythmic medications. (True/False)

7. A condition that involves a very rapid ventricular tachycardia is:

    a. Ventricular escape beat

    b. Ventricular flutter

    c. Ventricular aneurysm

    d. Ventricular hypertrophy

8. Which of the following is useful for detecting hypothermia

    a. Movement artefact

    b. Bradycardia

    c. Tachycardia

    d. Intraventricular conduction delay

9. The most obvious indicator of bilateral arm-leg reversal

    a. Flat line in Lead I

    b. Flat line in Lead III

    c. Inverted Lead I

    d. Upright aVR

10. Some ECG signs of this condition are the following: F waves in a saw-tooth pattern, 2 F waves for every QRS complex, and ventricular responses that have 3:1 or higher rates

    a. Atrial flutter

    b. AV block

    c. Junctional Escape Beats

    d. Bidirectional Ventricular Tachycardia

References

1. Surawicz, B. and Knilans, T., 2008. *Chou's Electrocardiography in Clinical Practice E-Book: Adult and Pediatric*. Elsevier Health Sciences.

2. Khan, E., 2004. Clinical skills: the physiological basis and interpretation of the ECG. *British journal of nursing*, *13*(8), pp.440-446.

3. Dubin, D., 2000. *Rapid interpretation of EKG's: an interactive course*. Cover Publishing Company.

4. Garcia, T.B., 2013. *12-lead ECG: The art of interpretation*. Jones & Bartlett Publishers.

5. Kusumoto, F.M., 2009. *ECG interpretation: from pathophysiology to clinical application*. Springer Science & Business Media.

6. Kors,J.A.,Macfarlane,P.,Mirvis,D.M.andPahlm,O.,2007.Recommendations for the standardization and interpretation of the electrocardiogram: part I: the electrocardiogram and its technology: a Scientific Statement from the American Heart Association Electrocardiography and Arrhythmias Committee, Council on Clinical Cardiology; the American College of Cardiology Foundation; and the Heart Rhythm Society. Endorsed by the International Society for Computerized Electrocardiology. *Heart Rhythm*, *4*(3), pp.394-412.

7. Hatala, R.A., Norman, G.R. and Brooks, L.R., 1997. The effect of clinical history on physician's ECG interpretation skills. In Advances in Medical Education (pp. 608-610). Springer, Dordrecht.

8. ***www.ecglibrary.com.*** Dean Jenkins and Stephen Gerred.

Answers to Exercises

Chapter 1

    1. B

    2. C

    3. False

    4. D

    5. 25

    6. half-standard

    7. 50

    8. C

    9. C

    10. False

Chapter 2

    1. C

    2. B

    3. C

    4. A

5. B

6. C

7. B

8. C

9. A

10. D

Chapter 3

1. A

2. B

3. C

4. D

5. E

6. A

7. C

8. C

9. D

10. B

Chapter 4

1. False

2. C

3. False

4. False

5. D

6. V3, V4

7. I, aVL, V5, V6

8. V1, V2

9. V1, V2, aVF

10. C

Chapter 5

1. B

2. C

3. A

4. A

5. A

6. False

7. B

8. A

9. A

10. A

Conclusion

Thank you again for buying this book!

I hope this book was able to help you to interpret the 12-Lead EKG/ECG. The next step is to study this book and other materials thoroughly.

You need to know as much as you can, so that you can provide the best care possible.

If you liked our book and you want to help us reach more people, please leave a review on Amazon.

Thank you and good luck with your medical career!

Join Our Community

Medical Creations is an educational company focused on providing study tools for Healthcare students.

We want to be as close as possible to our customers, that's why we are active on all the main Social Media platforms.

You can find us here:

www.facebook.com/medicalcreations

www.instagram.com/medicalcreations

www.twitter.com/medicalcreation (no 's')

www.pinterest.com/medicalcreations

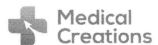

Kindle MatchBook

Kindle MatchBook is a feature that allows customers who have previously purchased a physical book from Amazon.com to receive the Kindle version for a discounted price or for free.

You can receive a copy of our EKG|ECG INTERPRETATION Kindle Edition for FREE.

Just go to the Kindle Version page of the book on Amazon and download the ebook.

Read your ebook on any device (phone, tablet, laptop).

Check Out Our Other Books

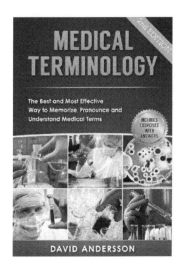

BEST SELLER ON AMAZON:

Medical Terminology:
The Best and Most Effective Way to Memorize,
Pronounce and Understand Medical Terms

Lab Values:
Everything You Need to Know about Laboratory
Medicine and its Importance in the Diagnosis of
Diseases

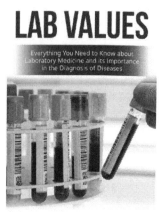

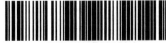

Made in the USA
San Bernardino, CA
25 February 2019